Walk a Mile in Our Shoes

By
Patricia A. Fisher

Published by
ITSMEEE™ Industries
Aurora, CO
USA

Walk a Mile in Our Shoes

Published by ITSMEEE™ Industries

All interior art by Patricia A. Fisher
Book layout and design by Patricia A. Fisher
Inside photography by Patricia A. and D.H. Fisher
Cover photography, book production and technical advice by D. H. Fisher
Cover production and design by
NZ Graphics, Lakewood, CO

Printed in the United States of America

First Edition

Library of Congress Control Number: 2004090710
Old ISBN: 0-9677231-4-0
New ISBN: 978-0-9677231-4-3

I would like to acknowledge the following people for their support and undying belief in the message of this book:

Dennis H. Fisher

Drs. William J. &
Mary E. Carder

Mr. Ron Markovich, LCSW

Martin Reichman, D.O.

Steve Henneman, M.A, LPC

Aurora Community
Mental Health Center

Other Titles by
Patricia A. Fisher

With Love ITSMEEE™
Copyright © 1997 by Patricia A. Fisher

With Love ITSMEEE™ II
Copyright © 1998 by Patricia A. Fisher

Introducing Number III, ITSMEEE™
Copyright © 1999 by Patricia A. Fisher

ITSMEEE™ On My Journey Home
Copyright © 1999 by Patricia A. Fisher
ITSMEEE™ Industries

Hello, ITSMEEE™ Again
Copyright © 2002 by Patricia A. Fisher
ITSMEEE™ Industries

ITSMEEE™ Beneath the Grey
An Autobiography
Copyright © 2003 by Patricia A. Fisher
ITSMEEE™ Industries

Other Titles (Continued)
By Patricia A. Fisher

From This Day Forward
Copyright © 2003 by Patricia A. Fisher
ITSMEEE™ Industries

I Want to LIVE!
Copyright © 2004 by Patricia A. Fisher
ITSMEEE™ Industries

Walk a Mile in Our Shoes
Copyright © 2005 by Patricia A. Fisher
ITSMEEE™ Industries

The Favor I Owe the World
Copyright © 2005 by Patricia A. Fisher
ITSMEEE™ Industries

Home Is Where We Park It!
Copyright © 2008 by Pat Fisher
Funhous Publishing

The Absence of Awful
Copyright © 2012 by Patricia A. Fisher
ITSMEEE™ Industries

Table of Contents:

Table of Contents Continued:

Interviews:

An Important Message:

ROSES ARE RED.

VIOLETS ARE BLUE.

THERE'S TWO OF ME,

AND ONE OF YOU…

Dear Reader Most Kind,

Tonight, I witnessed myself in fear. I had this huge dread of not being respected or loved.
Some fear is a good sign. It means I am no longer hiding. It means I am alive...

I have been crying, as I stay out here in a world of feelings and emotion. I have been tearfully shedding a few of my protective layers.

Passing away are the old and comfortable habits of necessity.
I am letting go of the resentment and judgment I put on myself and others.

I am no longer putting people in convenient, disarming, little categories.

I have forgiven the world, including myself, and I cry as the feelings wash over me.

My tears are like a constant baptism, and I am renewed and refreshed. I relax into a world of possibility, love and belonging, as I begin to give back the favor that I owe the world...

While writing this book, I decided to divide it into three sections:

1. My 'Journaling in Rhyme'
2. Interviews of Fellow Mental Health Consumers
3. Dear World

All three sections bring balance to "Walk a Mile in Our Shoes". They are in order so that the text is easier and more enjoyable to read.

I began publishing my writing seven years ago, hoping to be of assistance. I share my secrets in the name of love, respect, and truth. If you find a bit of humor, it would be frosting on the cake!

As you read on, you may be reminded that we humans are not so different from each other. 'Walk a Mile in Our Shoes' may help you see this for yourselves.

When we consumers of mental health, share our pain and joy, we know we are not alone. Almost every human being, is touched by pain and pleasure, and all the shades of grey in between.

One realization set me free more than any other. It was the knowledge that, while we are all miraculous beings, capable of much intelligence, we are all fallible and still only human.

Walk A Mile In Our Shoes

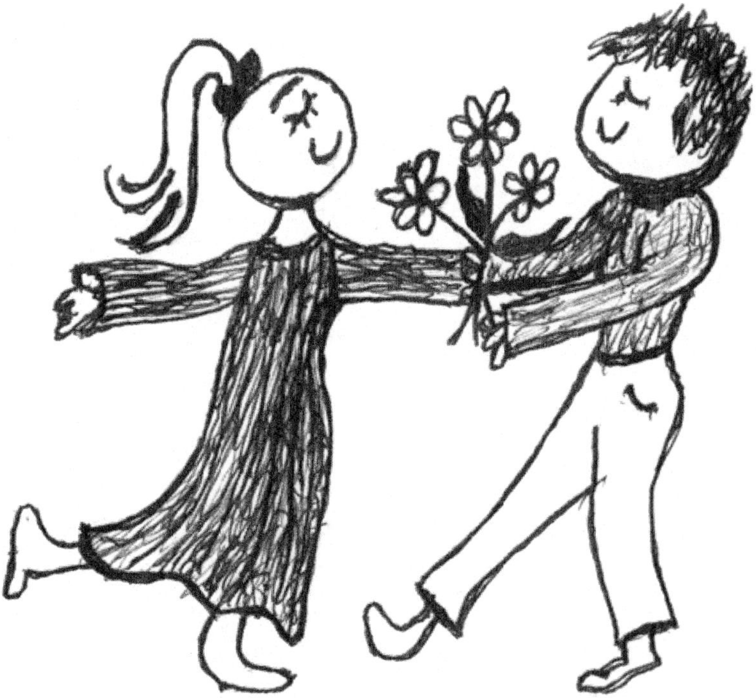

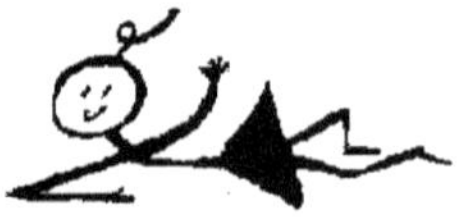

Marsha Kay DeChant

Born 6-27-1948
Passed on 9-23-2003

The following is a tribute to Marsha Kay DeChant. We could all learn a lesson from the way she lived.

Marsha was diagnosed with Multiple Sclerosis in 1976. She was bedridden for 14 long years. Yet she was an inspiration for anyone who had the good fortune of meeting her.

Her body slowly deteriorated, but her spirit stayed strong and vital.

I wrote 'Marsha's Little Secret' the day after I attended her funeral. It was an honor I won't forget. She was 55 years old.

Members of the family spoke of their thankfulness, that she is now free of that terrible physical bondage.

We spoke of her being in Heaven, and singing with her Dad, like she did in her youth.

I found myself basking in the love of our family. For, through marriage to 'my' Dennis, they are my family as well. Again, I am fortunate...

If you ever met her, you already know
'Marsha's Little Secret'.

Marsha's Little Secret

Oh, Marsha Kay,
What can I say?
A lot of us are blind.

We've got a lot
Of problems
Wearing on our mind.

We seem to search
For all those things
That we all
Think we need.

A lot of times
We're so afraid.
We're so afraid, indeed,

That we will miss
The very thing
That might give
Happiness

To all of us who worry
And speak of our
Distress.

We keep on searching
All the years
That we are on
This Earth.

We try to find
That 'something'
To tell us of
Our worth.

Oh, is it gold,
Dear Marsha Kay?
Fine stones
That sparkle bright?

Like stars
Up in the heavens,
That light the sky
At night?

Could it be
Fine linens,
Or silk against
Our skin,

Or other fine and
Lovely cloth
To comfort us
Within?

Or some of us
Buy houses,
As fine as they
Can be,

So far beyond
Our budget,
Yes, some
Outrageous fee!

Marsha Kay,
All that it took,
Right from
The very start,

Was hidden
In your smile,
And sheltered
In your heart.

You gave it
Oh, so freely.
'Twas there
For us to take.

It wasn't
Gold or silver.
We'd make a
Huge mistake,

If we met
Our Marsha,
And we remained
So blind,

That we did not
See riches
Within her smile
So kind.

The Bible speaks
Of many things
That come from
Up above.

Marsha's little secret was,
"The best of these
Is love"...

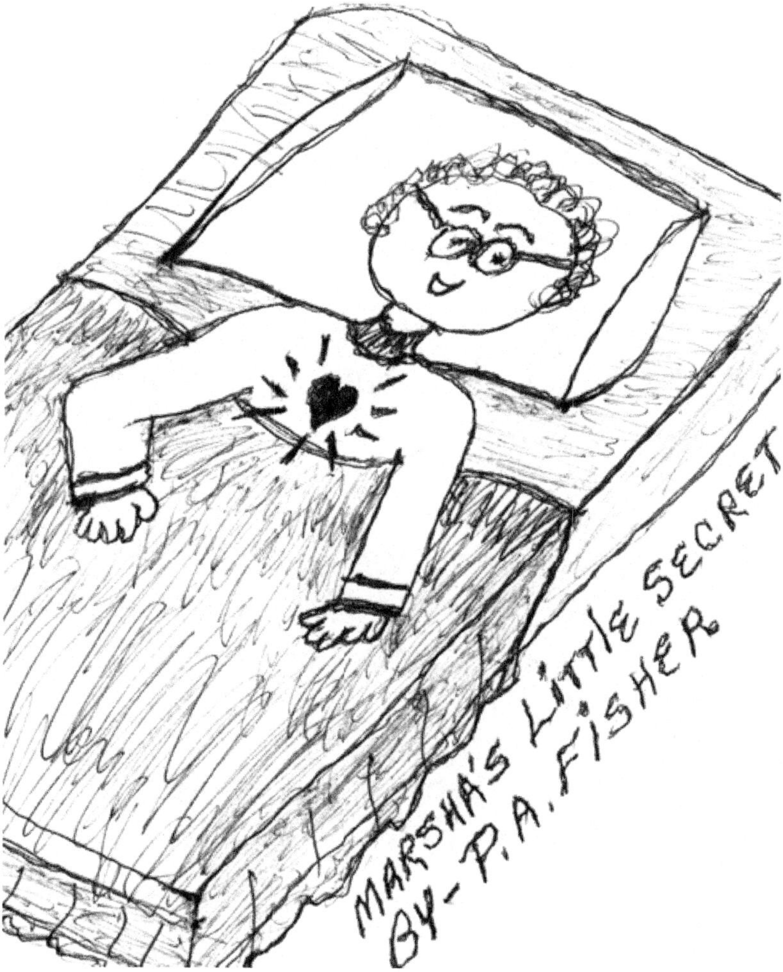
MARSHA'S Little SECRET
BY- P.A. FISHER

Dearest Heavenly Father

Today is Dennis and my 30th anniversary. We spoke our vows a second time, right here in our motor home. No one else was here except us.

There were no dollars spent, no invitations sent out, and no gifts necessary.

We spoke of our amazing love for each other. We spoke of the next 30 years, and we promised, again, that we will be together for an eternity...

Thank you, God, for coming to the ceremony. It was lovely...

The Two of Us

For you, the man I married,
For you, who picked up the
slack,

For you, who gave me love,
Not always getting it back.

You've been my shining star
Through dark and dismal times.

For you have shown me love,
Not only with nickels and dimes.

You've shown it by hearing my
words.
So often you understand.

The kind of love you give
Is the kind with an open hand.

You always love with your
actions.
So often, people do not.

The example that you set
Simply cannot be bought!

You've shown it by fixing a light.
Or changing a battery,

Or by doing lots of things,
And not needing flattery.

These things are like special gifts
All of a sudden found,

When I walk into a room,
Where he's put on some sound.

It's when I least expect
Something good for me.

I suddenly see no garbage,
But no clean bag I see...!

I gripe about the bag,
Completely ignoring his plight.

You can guess what happens.
We get into a fight!

It's when I'm feeling bored,
Or maybe feeling low,

He's turned on the television
At the start of my favorite show.

He's been known to do the dishes.
One hand can count the times!

"That's one thing that Pat must do.
Dishwater's awful," he whines.

He's very rarely angry.
He's slow to judge anyone.

He's very, very practical,
And yet he's loads of fun.

He tells me something off the
wall.
It takes me off my guard.

I laugh for such a long, long
while.
He can be such a card!

So back a ways, when we first
met,
I guess I had much to learn.

Most of the folks I didn't trust.
To Dennis, I started to turn.

Through the years we lived it all.
We went through tons of pain!

But happiness was accessible.
Sometimes it fell like rain!

No garbage bag, nor dishes done,
Nor wiping off a table,

They're very insignificant,
As long as I am able.

If we had a yacht,
Or our own private jet,

Or my cosmetic surgery,
(I'm gonna get a new set)!

If I had a million,
Or art extraordinaire,

Or all the precious jewelry,
And tailored clothes to wear!

If we bought an island,
We'd more than measure up,

To all the Rockefellers!
(We must fill our cup)!

We'd fly to Bora-Bora
Whenever we felt blue.

To dinner with the president-
Six hundreds bucks for two!

We'd take our trips to Africa.
Safari's are quite the thing!

But they don't compare to 'my'
Dennis.
'Cause he makes my heart sing'!

The treasures of which I have spoken,
Would be empty objects for me,

If I were without 'my' Dennis,
He's most important to me.

A person needs somebody
With whom to laugh and cry.

Without these things we're poor,
Until the day we die.

I learned very much about love.
I learned to give it in turn.

I started showing the love that I felt.
"Say it with actions," I learned...

Now, when he walks to one of
the rooms,
He sees a little surprise.

Instead of seeing plain old me,
I've Mascara on my eyes!

He looks from me around the
room.
Someone had cleaned up the
place.

I look at him, and start to brag.
(I guess I still need praise).

Now we pitch in to do our part.
Now we get so much done!

I love how we both are standing
tall—
Two people, and yet only one...

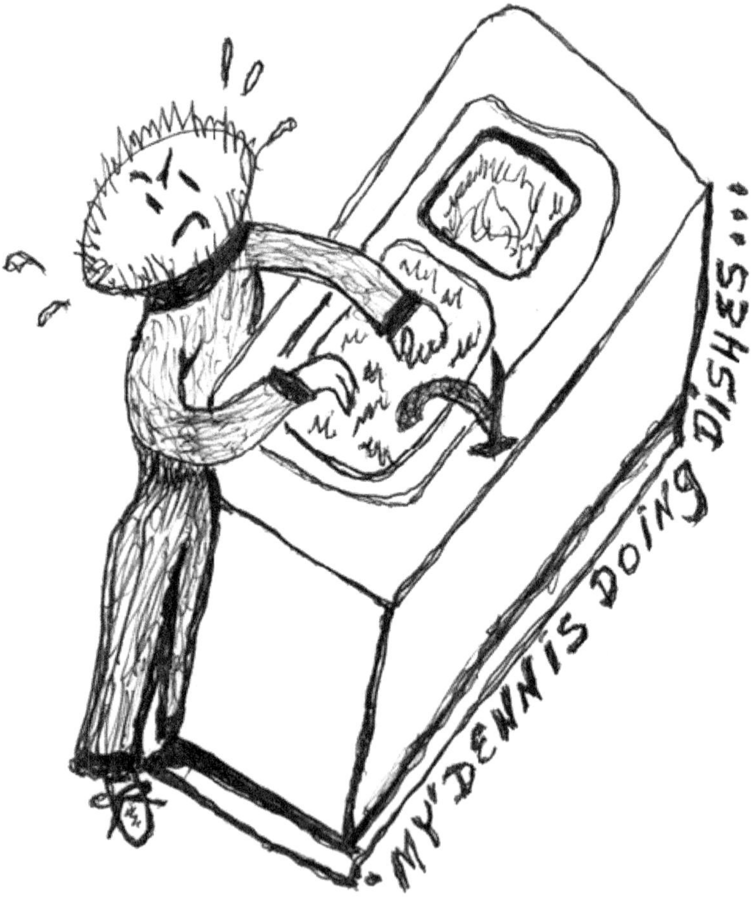
MY DENNIS DOING DISHES...

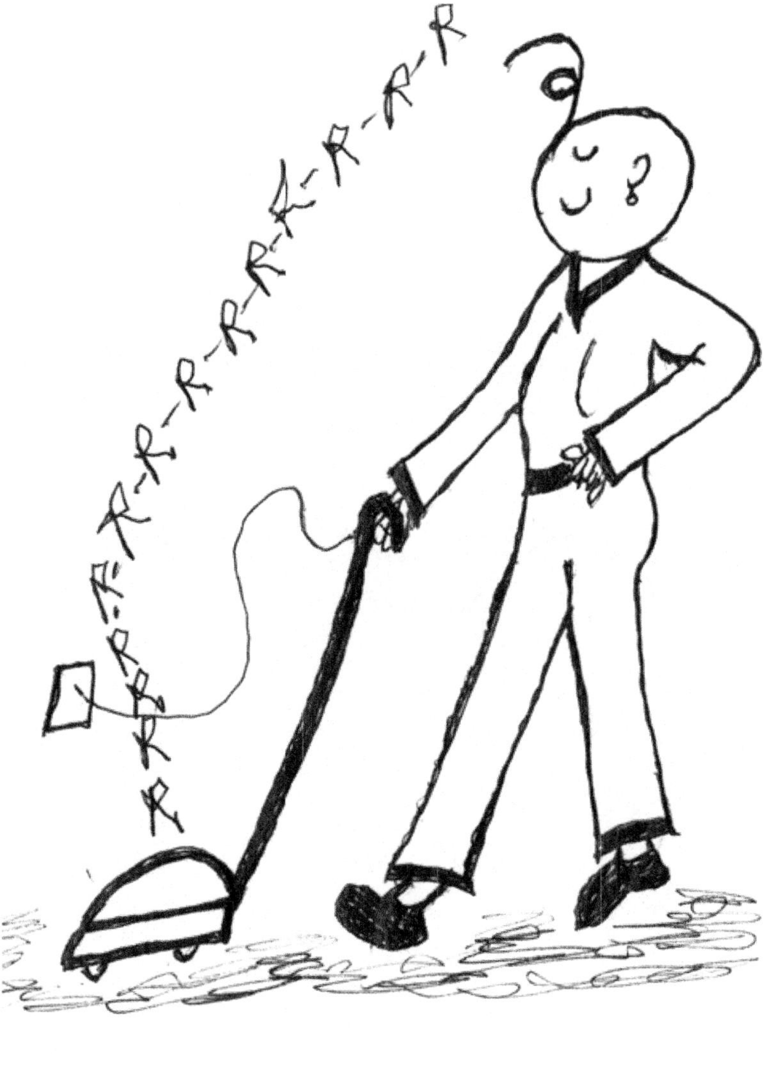

I DON'T GO BACK ON
MY WORD.

I JUST CHANGE MY
MIND.

WHEN SOMEONE ASKS ME, "ARE YOU GOING TO DO SOMETHING?"

TO GET OFF THE HOOK, I LIKE TO ANSWER,

"IT ALL DEPENDS ON WHETHER I DO OR NOT!"

Daddy shared that he once had an accident in his car.

He said that he didn't have any idea how he ended up in a ditch. He swore he had been following the street's white line.

Finally, he said, through a grin, that he had been following a skunk by mistake...

Another time,
we were driving to
Mexico in Daddy’s car.

He called back to us,
“If you guys get
scared during the
drive, you can close
your eyes, ‘cause
that’s what I’m going
to do!”

When people appear to
be aggravated for no
apparent reason,

They usually just need
a little more love...

Mom

Oh My God, I'm My Mother!

With Mom at work, and my Dad gone, I spent my early years with little guidance. The next 30-40 years were spent undoing all of my confusion...

At 55, I now am realizing that my Mother was smarter and stronger than I ever knew.

Instead of cringing, when someone notices our similarities, I feel grateful and honored.

Instead of being in shock, and wishing there wasn't any likeness between us, I find myself thanking God for my ever knowing her at all!

We spent hours on the phone.
Someone asked what we talked
about for so much time!

I was speechless! I had no idea!

Finally, the only words that came
to mind, were at the beginning
of our every call. I get a bit
melancholy thinking back to the
millions of times I sang out to
her, "Hi Mom, ITSMEEE...!"

I no longer exclaim,
"Oh My God, I'm My Mother!"

Now days, I whisper softly to my
higher power,

"Thank you God.
I'm a lot like Mom..."

Mama's Rolling Pin

My Mama had
A rolling pin.

She was
So very wise,

But then she had
A heart attack,

While baking
Her great pies.

It happened
In September-

A sad
And angry day.

I look back
And remember,

And I get sad
This way.

In her own
Apartment

She rolled out
All her dough,

Like many times
Before this.

I want us all
To know.

On September
Eleven,

In her private
Home,

She heard
The news

On her
TV,

While we were
On the phone.

She then spoke of
Her weakness

That happened
From the shock.

Her heart
Just couldn't take it.

'Twas hard
For her to walk.

Other
Complications

Began to
Get her down,

But she was real
Courageous,

And faith
Is what she found.

Since then,
She passed away.

It started
On that day,

That day
Back in September,

The eleventh,
I remember.

While going
Through her stuff,

A project
That was tough,

I wanted things
Of hers for me-

Some for just
A memory.

Then I opened
Up a drawer,

And what I felt
Was strange.

Her rolling pin
Was lying there,

And this,
I could not change.

I left it lying
In the drawer.

It touched me to
My very core.

At the time
I could not see

The value
Of that pin to me.

I've thought of it
So many times.

I've realized
Within these Rhymes.

The pain and loss
Of my dear Mom,

Was caught within
My front of calm.

Then tears I shed
So openly.

That pin meant
Oh so much to me.

'Twas the beginning
Of the end.

For my sweet Mama
Could not mend.

A little old lady
With a grin

Was Mama
And her rolling pin.

Innocently
Making pies,

A heart attack,
And then she dies...

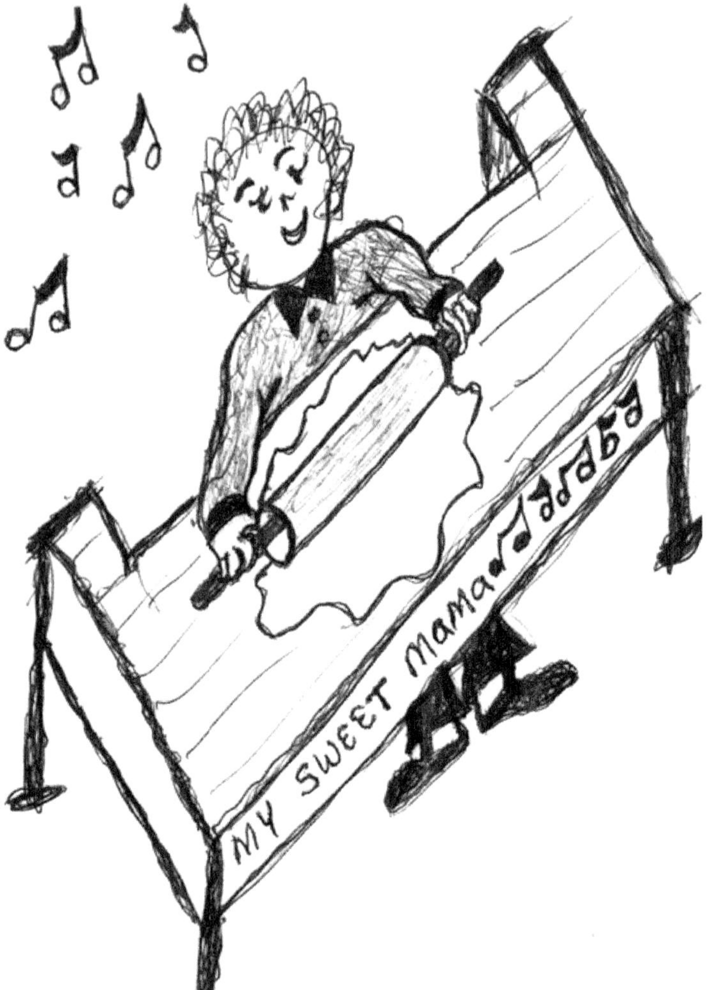
MY SWEET Mama

Mama's Little Gesture

My Mom, Dennis, and I were on one of our many outings. This time it just happened to be Barnum and Bailey's Circus.

We had a great time seeing the elephants, acrobats, lion tamers and all the other wonderful parts of 'The Greatest Show on Earth'.

When we started to go home, we worked our way through the noisy crowds.

Finally, we were inside the car. I slowly started backing out of our parking space, and noticed some people behind us to the right.

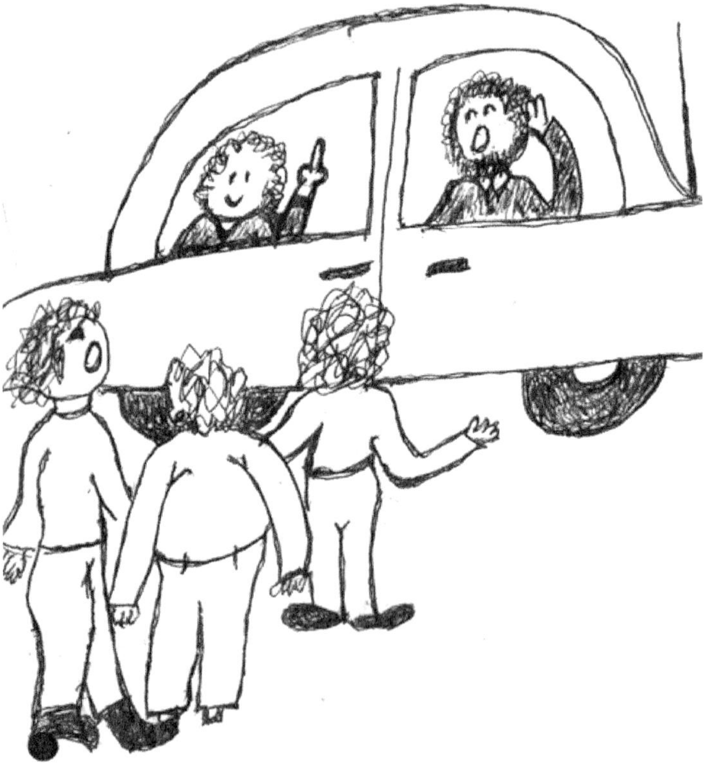

I backed up a little bit more, as they waited in irritation.

This is when my 70 year old Mother threw them 'the finger'!

We were all quite shocked. The people, now beside the car, didn't know how to react. Their mouths dropped open in disbelief. Their faces told us that they never expected to see what this little, white haired lady had done.

I smile, as I look back. For the three of us giggled almost all the way home.

As far as I know, it was the first and last occurrence of 'Mama's Little Gesture'.

My Mama's Legacy

I thought that you were weak,
That you were not as strong,

As anyone I met.
How could I be wrong?

Seventy seven years,
Of life upon this earth,

Giving all you had,
Starting at your birth.

Mom, I could not see,
Clear enough to know,

How great and strong you were,
Since many years ago.

Though you've passed away,
I want for you to know,

That you are now my mentor,
And that I love you so.

You really made a difference
In my life don't you see?

You changed this wounded
planet.
You changed not only me.

You have caused much more
Than a ripple in life's ocean,

Not only having daughters,
But I think you were chosen

By a higher power,
To show us how to be

A warrior on this planet.
This is what I see.

Thanks for my initiative,
And power to go on.

For I'm a warrior, also.
Each day I must be strong.

You are an inspiration.
I look back through your life.

You laughed between the
heartaches.
For you had pain and strife.

But God gave you some babies,
And you were really thrilled.

For this was all you wanted.
This made your life fulfilled.

Well, here's one of your
daughters,
Happy, I must say,

To hear somebody tell me,
"You're like your Mom today."

Can We Have It All?

My love,
We have been wounded.
This earth
Where we came from,

Brings challenge
So gigantic,
And yet
We've had some fun.

I'm twenty years
Your senior.
Inside of me
You've seen,

Equality
And value,
A fellow human being.

You do not
Hide your light
In order
To fit in.

Your truth
Shines very brightly.
I don't
Remember when,

I've seen
Another like you,
Or felt them
Loving me.

My heart says
There is goodness
Between us.
Don't you see?

I guess
I've never felt this
From someone
Quite so young.

We both
Respect each other.
Equality
Is fun!

Neither of us better.
Neither of us less.
I am now beginning
To learn, I do confess.

That we are both
Quite different.
This I celebrate!

Uniqueness is
A gift from God.
It's value
Is quite great.

Let's shine our light
As brightly,
As we have
All this time.

For there is
Just one Tanya-
For sure,
One of a kind.

We both made an
Arrangement
That we would
Share our truth.

Even when
It's painful,
Our friendship
Is the proof.

For we can
Laugh and play.
A balance,
It can be.

Can we have
It all?
Well, let's just
Wait and see...

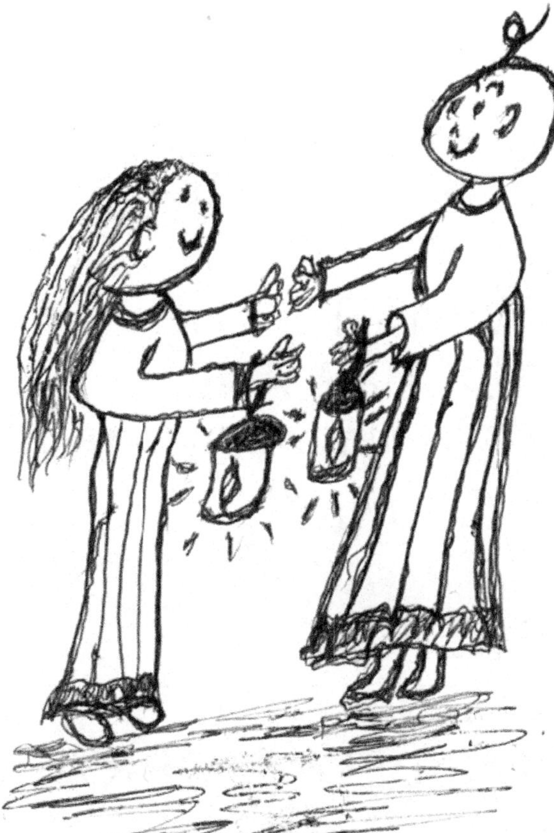

A PERSON, WITH A MENTAL ILLNESS, WAS WATCHING A FOOTBALL GAME.

HE WENT TO THE SNACK BAR AND ASKED, "DO YOU HAVE ANY CASHEWS?"

THE PERSON WORKING THERE ANSWERED, "SORRY, WE DON'T SERVE NUTS..."

"I'M GOING TO BEAT YOU UP," SAID THE NIMROD!

"OH YEAH! YOU AND WHAT ARMY," SAID THE WINGNUT!

"MY RIGHT 'ARMIE' AND MY LEFT 'ARMIE'," SAID THE NIMROD...

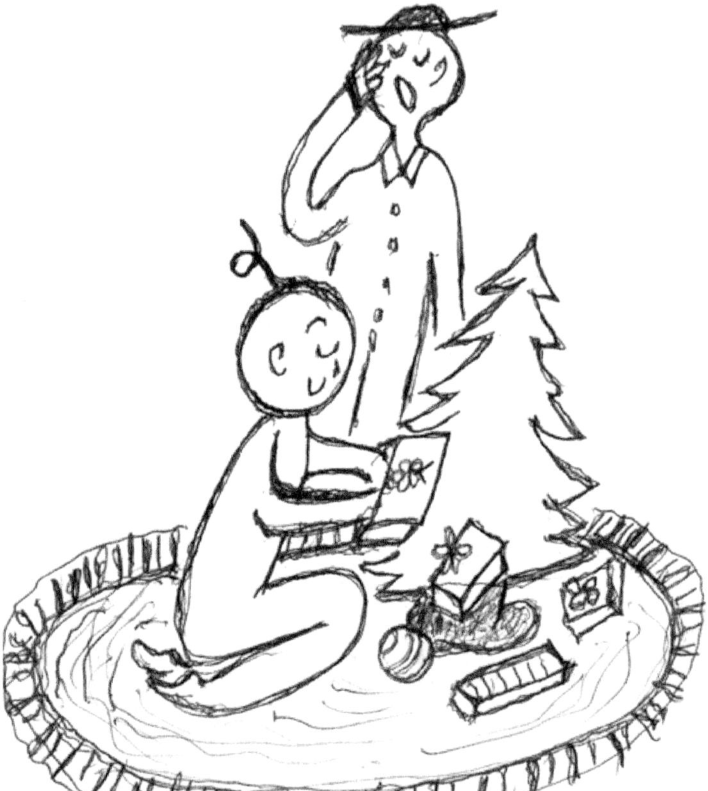

What Is the Power of Presence? (Or Is It Presents)?

Dearest Kate,

It is Christmas time again, and I find myself in wonder of its mysteries. Your question has had me on an inward voyage, causing me to again search my heart for answers.

Within me is the magic of love, and the closeness of family and friends. I count the ways we openly choose to show good will toward each other.

'My' Dennis and I like to share our home and abundance.

We give gifts to many, many people. This keeps us buying in moderation, when shopping for 'tokens of our love'...

We feel that a carefully chosen remembrance, of each person, is much better than spending a huge amount of money and going into debt.

Yet, when we fix a big meal, with love in our hearts, we share ourselves in another way. For some reason, having people over to our home, is like receiving the greatest gift of all.

Is not love the tie that binds?

To see how we transform ourselves, at this time of year, is a miracle in itself.

It appears that we are closer to our Higher Power, and our eyes begin to sparkle brighter from the light we cradle within.

What's most important? Is it the presence of ourselves, or is it the presents that we wrap?

I feel they both have their place. For there can be love in each one.

The Higher Power, I believe in, felt a lot of joy when he created material things. These were not only the embodiment of Human Beings, but the big and little treasures we all share.

And so, little Kate, from my heart to yours, the power of each is the same. For the power of each comes from love...

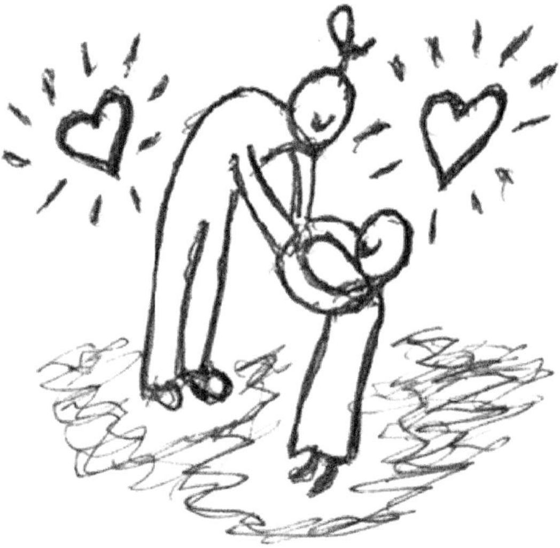

DISTANCING

CAN

CAUSE

JUST AS MUCH

FEELING

AS BEING

VERY, VERY CLOSE...

My Friend is a Breast Cancer Survivor...

(And Author of, "Dreamwalk"
By Rachael Clearwater)

My friend's a real survivor.
My friend from long ago,
Shows signs of some nirvana.
It's rare when she feels low.

She's happy and she's thankful.
Reminding me of what?
Reminding me of happiness
Away down in her gut.

She came so close to dying,
But more than this she bore.
They just defiled her body.
She could not handle more.

They pushed her far beyond the
mark, that she drew for herself.
Only life was her request,
And all that she deemed wealth.

With Love and Laughter
For 35 years,
Your friend,
Patricia A. Fisher
(Pat)

MY MOM AND DAD

MADE

A

'PATSY'

OUT OF ME!

SHOULD'VE DIDN'T MAKE IT

My Blessings

Dear Heavenly Father,
They told me not to pray!
I said, "Dear Lord, My God,
They stole my words away!"

They said it was against the law!
I can no longer thank,

My Dear Heavenly Father
Whose blood in grace I drank.

The self same God who's in my
Heart,
I thank Him for my life!

He wants from me
Great things you see--

Things learned from pain
And strife!

I will share all that I know,
And show you how I live.

I stay close to the Father,
My life to Him I give.

You might call me a Christian—
Even when I'm down.

Through valley of death
I talk to Him
Until I'm safe and sound...

Sins don't mean we're
'Less than'
That our worth is quite small,

For, since I met Our Father,
I'm standing very tall.

Our Father loves His children.
We don't need to fret!

He doesn't want us,
'Less than',
Or feeling so upset.

He wants to love His children,
And give us what we need.

A lot is done, when someone
Says,
"Goodbye, Go with God's speed".

No one knows how fast,
God's speed, alas, can be!

I just know it doesn't hurt.
It's not too fast for me.

Nor is it so very slow
That we just can't slow down.

God is good. He cuddles us,
And keeps us Heaven bound.

He would not want us all
Ashamed.
He says we are His treasure.

I think The Ten Commandments
May be His only measure.

He uses it to tell us
Just how well we did,

From somewhere up in Heaven,
Since we were just a kid...

PEOPLE MAY NOT
REMEMBER EXACTLY
WHAT YOU *DID*, OR
WHAT YOU *SAID*,

BUT THEY WILL
ALWAYS REMEMBER
HOW YOU MADE THEM
FEEL.

(Author Unknown)

This Little Spark

I 'hit a little bump' here lately.
Hell describes it pretty well.

Sometimes my world changes,
and becomes hostile. Sometimes
I don't see the world as mine.

But it appears that, during all
the hell and suffering, there is
this little spark inside me.

It seems to stay lit, awaiting an
hour, a minute, or day, that life
becomes good.

These are the times I live for
and cherish. These are the times
of relief. These are the times
when I celebrate life.

Finding Our Uniqueness

As I sit here, I am living, loving, and believing...

God is so good! He speaks to me through people who embrace their own uniqueness.

I am fortunate to have a husband, who is also my dear friend.

We have shared our lives for all these years, and I don't know anyone like him.

As of April 2002, I have known the peace of a closer relationship with God.

Yet, I still find myself choosing between two different realities.

Which world will I choose? Or is there only one world—one world where we all get along and see each other as special?

There are some things I can't share by speaking, so they end up within the pages of my literary creations.

My books are a safe way for me to share, and a safe way for others to hear me.

They read my words in the privacy of their own space. Most of the time, they like what they read, and they let me know...

This is at last, my joy and my freedom! I never knew who I was, until my thoughts started spilling over onto the pages.

I found myself by reading what I, myself, wrote.

The wheels grind slowly, and there is a lot of waiting. I would like to speak to the whole world.

Changing one person's life is very vital, but this just shows me how amazing it would be to reach millions!

If I could help millions to experience their uniqueness, it would be millions of times the joy for me.

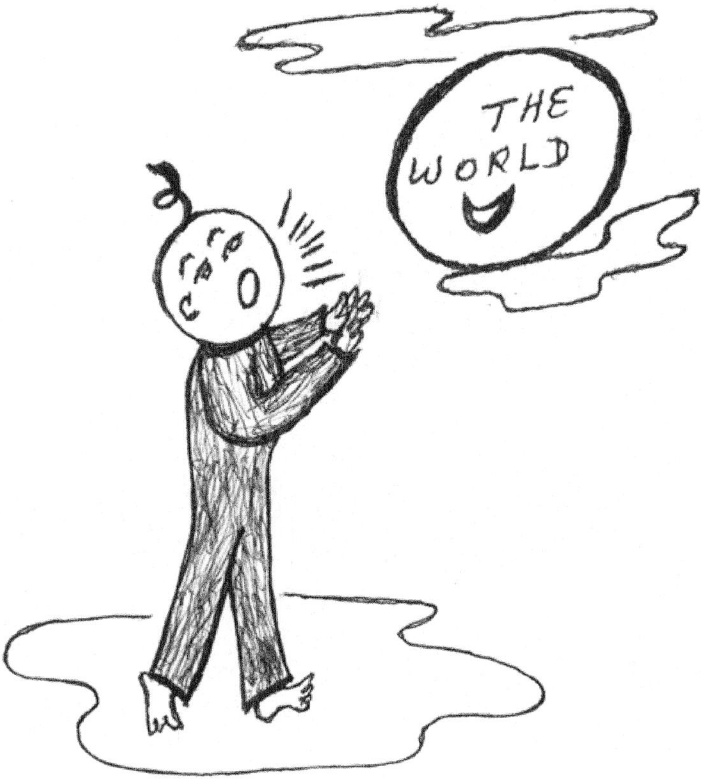
THE
WORLD

I'd like to be around, as all these people, take on this knowledge, that they make a difference— that there is no other person on earth exactly like them— and that the universe needs them just the way they are!

The earth would be full of people celebrating their differences, instead of fighting with each other because of them.

Each morning they would awaken, with a little smile on their face, and a renewed anticipation of what the day might hold for them...

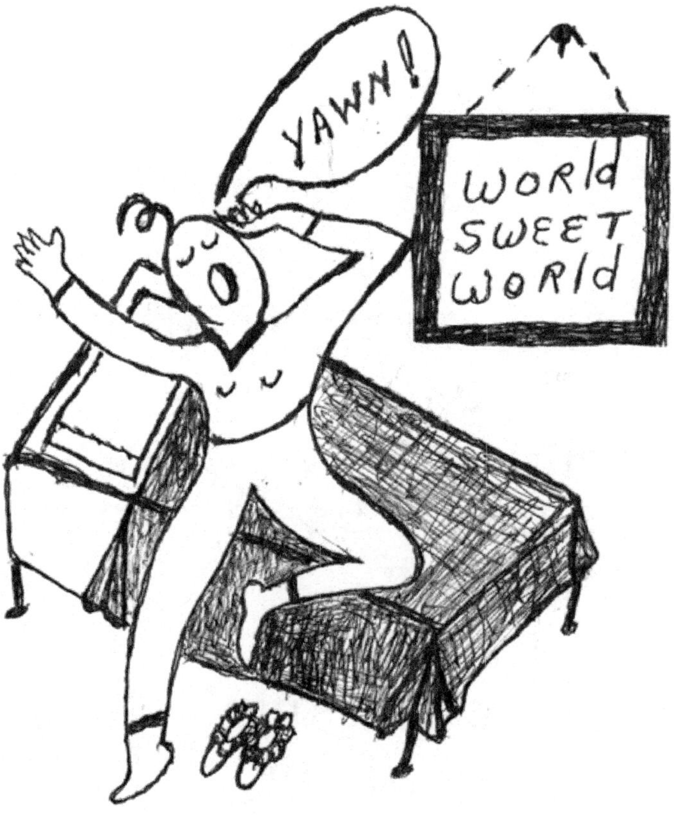
YAWN!
WORLD
SWEET
WORLD

Our four-year-old niece, Shantel and I, were sitting at the top of the stairs.

She saw a picture of me from a long time ago. I was in a bikini.

She exclaimed, "Who is that?" I said, "That's me."

She didn't understand, and cried out, "WHAT HAPPENED?"

This minister painted his church.

After two sides, he thinned the paint with water. He thinned it more than once.

When he was finished, he stood back admiring his work.

He then heard a loud voice that said, "Repaint and thin no more!" (Author unknown)

A Part of Ourselves

We parked our R.V. at a rest area in Arkansas. We slept among some big, noisy, 18 wheelers, and other R.V.s.

The sign said, "overnight camping only." Dennis and I had never heard of camping at a rest stop, and we were pleased.

We were dressed before day-break with coffee in hand. How fun it was cruising down I-40 before dawn!

After a couple of hours, we spotted an animal on the side of the road.

It was a beautiful little puppy! His eyes met mine, and I swear he smiled at me!

We couldn't turn our rig around for about 10 miles. When we finally did, there he was, right back at mile marker 190!

I was so excited!

We both fell in love with him immediately. We tried to lure him to us by offering food, and cooing noises.

He'd leap toward us, bark frantically, and run away. He seemed to be playful, but very much afraid, at the same time...

Then, we called a nearby town. There was no listing for animal control, so we called the police.

Soon, a patrolman drove up. He tried to hand a piece of bologna to our frisky friend.

Nope! Not interested!

I asked the officer about a tranquilizer gun, or some other way of catching an animal. He said, "We usually just do nothing. This pup has been out here for three days."

By this time, I was in tears. I felt this tiny life being torn away. I'd felt this way only once before, and now I was feeling it again.

Nothing more could be done, so we were urged to get back in our motor home.

We reluctantly drove away, knowing we were leaving behind a part of ourselves.

There was one last thing I had to do. I called police dispatch again. The same girl answered the phone.

I announced who we were, and said, "You know that puppy we wanted to take with us? We wanted to take care of him, take him to a Vet, and make him part of our family.

He was just too scared to come close, so we're on our way home.

No matter what happens, we just wanted you to know, we named him Freeway..."

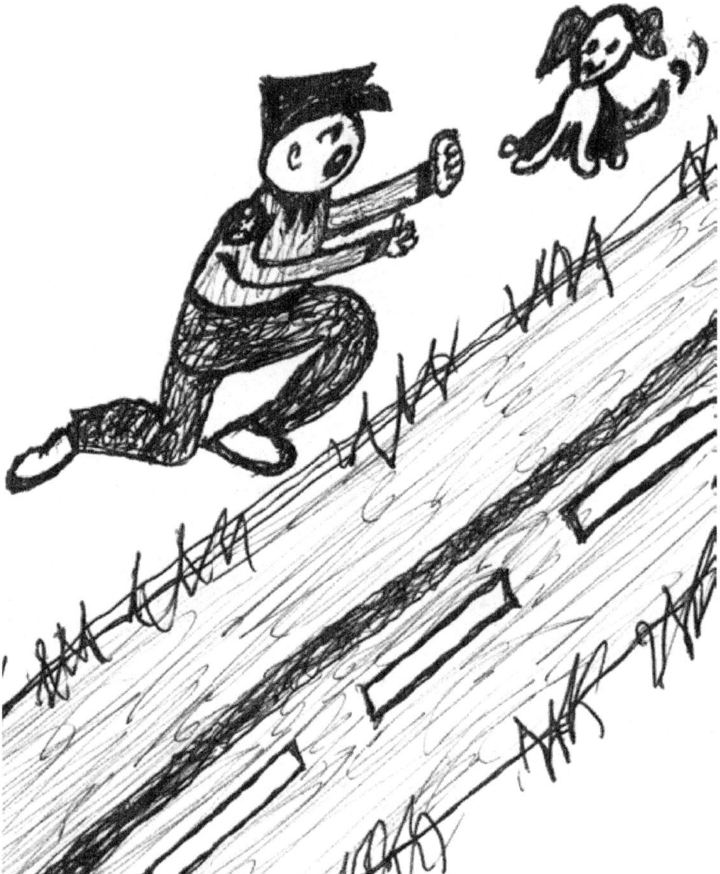

We were in Yuma, Arizona. I told 'my' Dennis that I really liked the place!

He remarked, "You must have a sense of Yuma..."

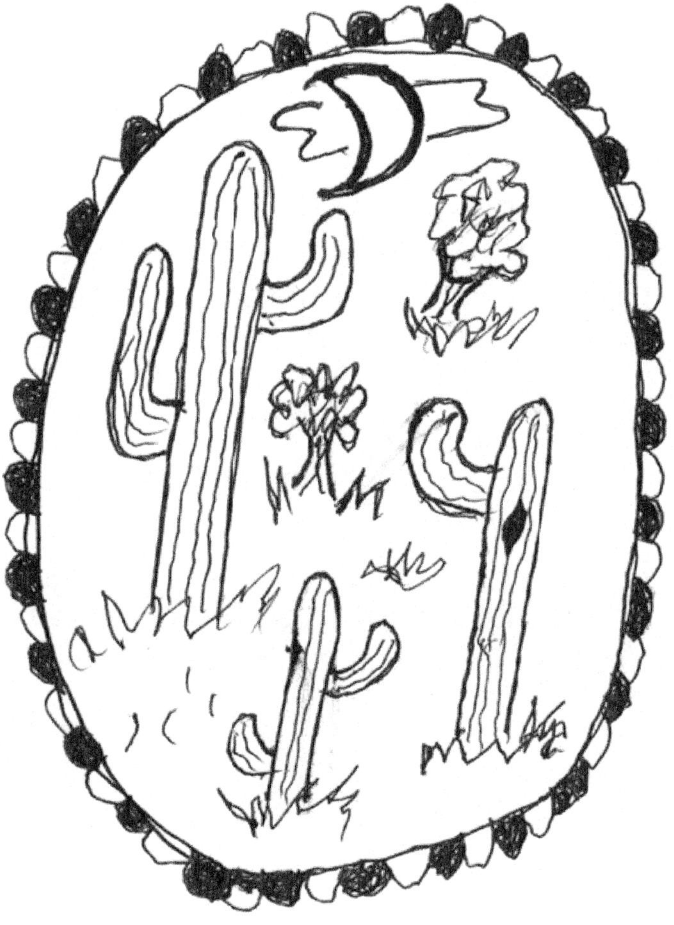

Ohio Hills

We were driving along, looking
at Ohio's beautiful scenery.

The lush hills boasted of
incredible reds, warm oranges,
and the rich browns and greens
of Fall.

My husband said,
"Look over there on that hill! It's
so beautiful!"

I told him, "We must have come
here just for the hill of it."

CONSTANTLY
BEHAVING IN A WAY
YOU CAN BE PROUD
OF

HELPS KEEP YOU
FROM BEING
AFFECTED BY OTHER
PEOPLE'S *STUFF.*

('My Dennis')

Nicholas

I have a six foot comrade—
Maybe six foot plus.

He's such a good
And humble man,
Walking among us.

When he was born,
He was so cute,
And smart as he could be.

He'd make us smile
At things he did,
When he was only three.

Remembering
His growing years
Still fails me at this time.

I know that we
Spent Christmas

At his house—
Oh so fine!

He grew up
A little more.
He became a man.

Still with problems,
Deep within.
I think I understand...

Divorce came
Between his folks.

Later,
His Dad died!

I don't know
If Nicholas
Ever even cried.

He's 30 years
Of age now,
Still searching for some peace.

I would bet
A part of him
Still wants the pain to cease.

Sweet Nicholas
Go back there.
Embrace your child self.

No use to keep
That part of you
Just sitting on a shelf.

I believe,
Dear Nicholas,
This child part of you,

Is causing
Pain and anguish.
Yes, I believe it's true.

Go back
My little comrade,
To where your pain was great.

Cry the tears,
And feel the rage.
It still is not too late.

This child self
Needs love from you.
For he is incomplete.

The older Nick
Needs closure.
One day you both will meet.

So sweet
Will be your feelings.

So calm
When you have said,

Everything you need to,
Words that you may dread.

After all has settled,
And peace is in that place,

Where no more rage
Abides in you—
Just smiles on your face,

Your life will be more peaceful.
More time will be spent glad.

Face your loss
Of long ago,
And say goodbye to Dad...

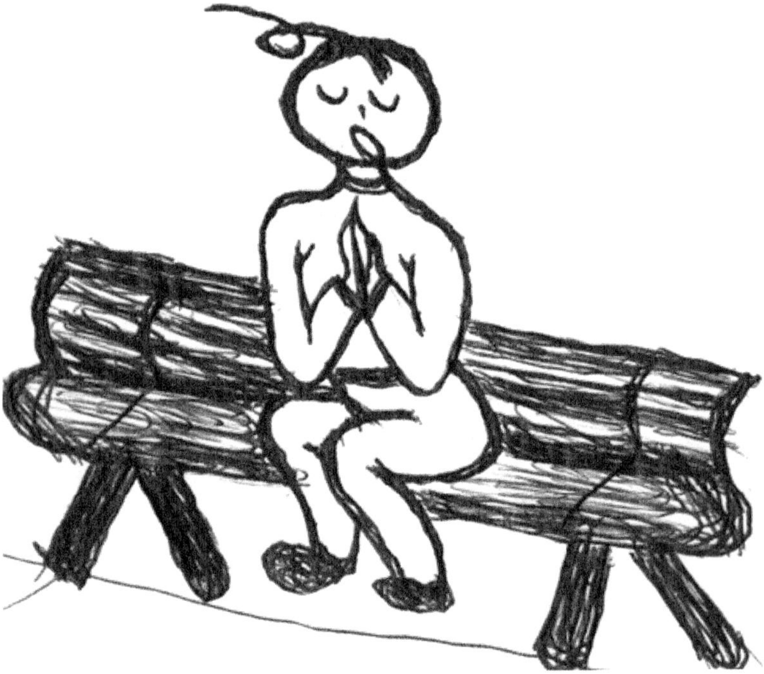

God, Don't Take Me Now

Nope, not yet, I have
To stay.

I have a lot to do
Today!

I need more time
On this old earth,

To share the light
Of my rebirth.

Good morning, God!
What can I say?
You're who makes me
Feel this way.

Your holy spirit
Washed me clean.

Since that day,
On you, I lean.

My prayers are answered
'Fore they're said.

I speak to God
(My daily bread).

Yes, each day,
First thing at morn,

I thank the Lord
That I was born.

Just to feel,
And be alive,

Or just to make it,
And survive,

Makes me thankful,
Makes me free,

Makes me feel
Just heavenly!

Dearest Father,
Up above,

May your children
Know of love.

May they turn
This love within.

Then forgive
Themselves of sin.

They're just human.
Let them know.

Such acceptance
Helps them grow.

I will help
This world, I vow!

Please, dear God,
Don't take me now!

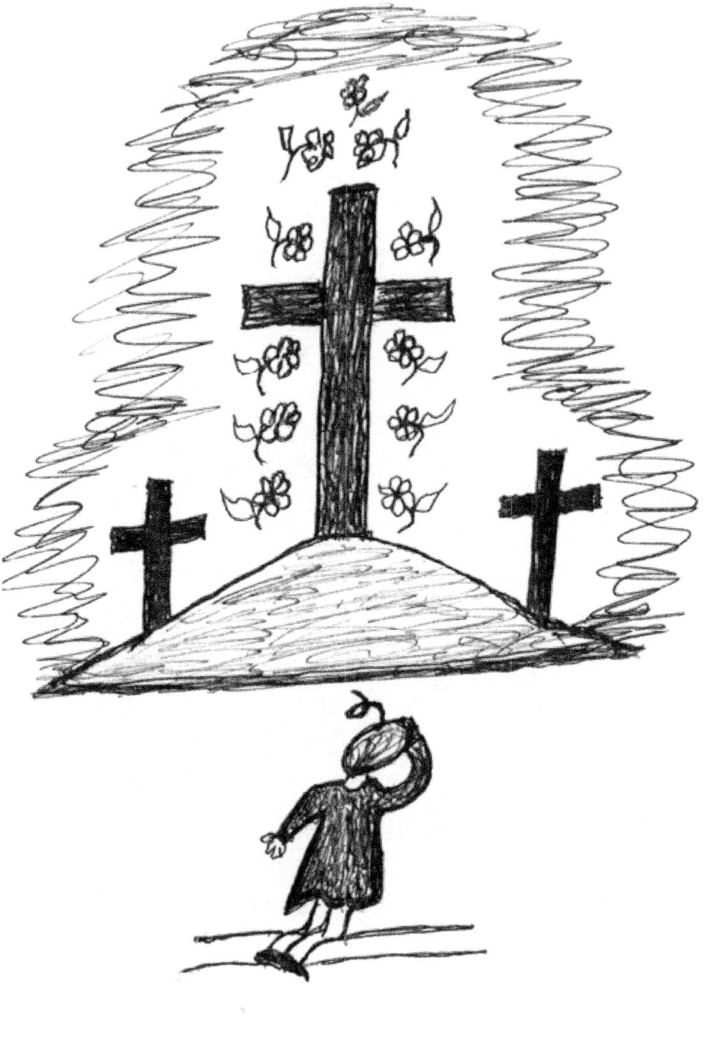

Patricia A. Fisher

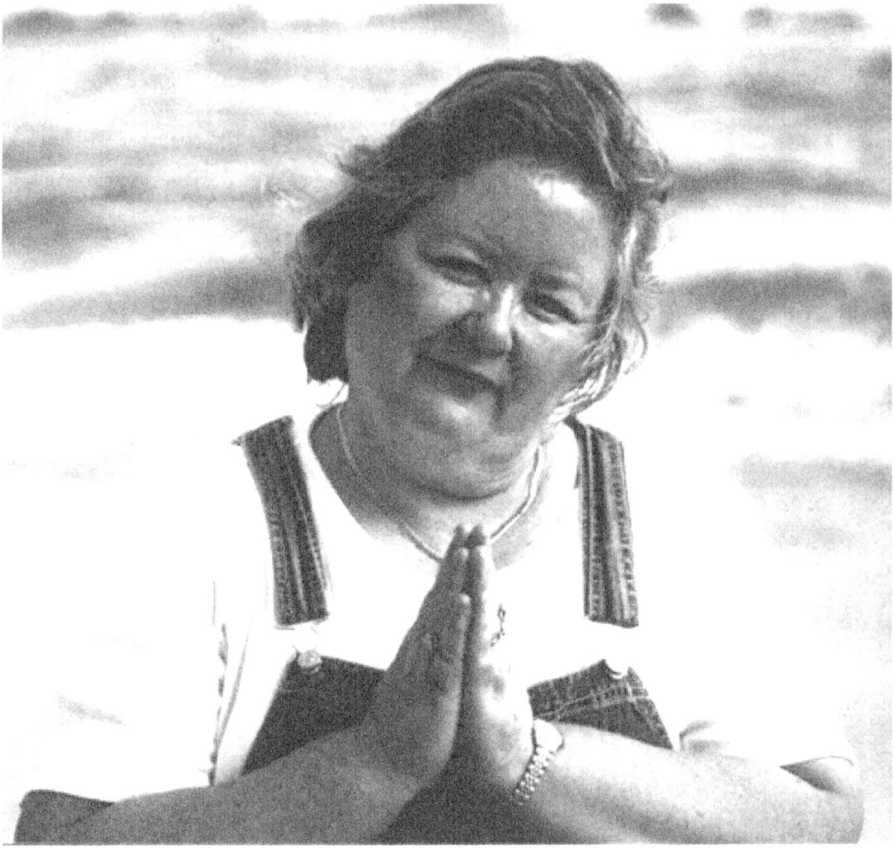

Thank you
for being
a part of
Our
~~My~~
Journey...
Patricia A.
Fisher

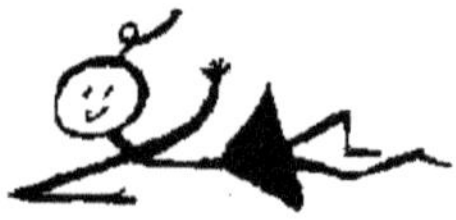

What Is Your Story?

Interviews of Fellow Mental Health Consumers

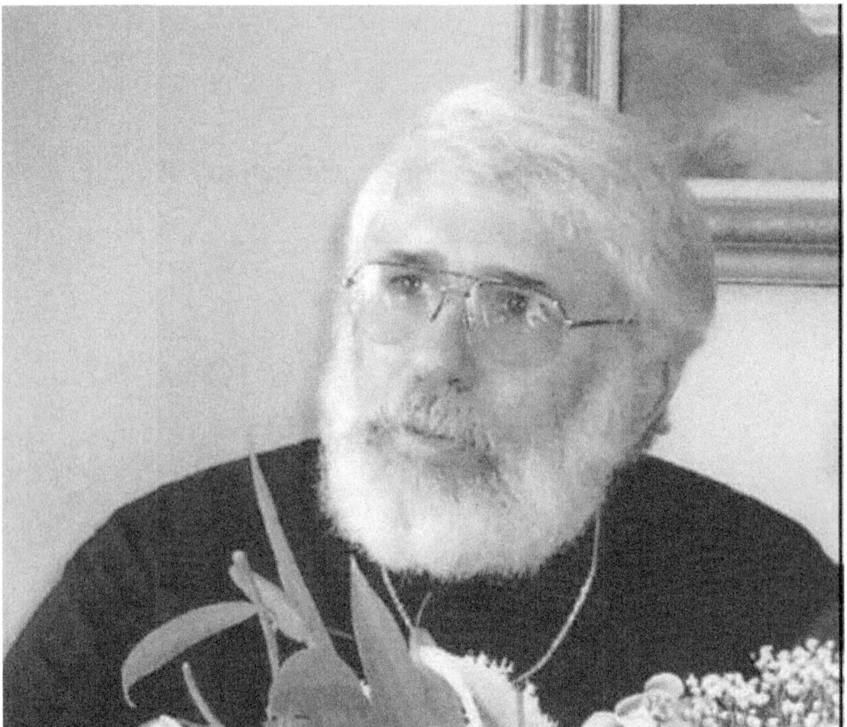

From a photo by Kate

D. H. Fisher
What Is Your Story?

What are 3 things that keep you going while you are in the pits?

I change the subject by finding something to do that I think I can do, and I push forward with that—even though I don't feel like doing anything! At times, this only takes the edge off.

At other times, it turns me all the way around. When I forge ahead, and ignore the feelings, I then find enjoyment and I get really involved!

What are 3 things you do to stay out of the pits?

The main thing for me is to stay busy! Another is leaving the house, if I'm uncomfortable there. (Change environment)
I can think of only two...

Tell me something about your past -- anything that comes to your mind.

Overall my past was pretty positive. It's kind of difficult to answer that... I had really good working relationships, and I've been lucky in love. I guess I've had a pretty good life.

What happened to bring on your affliction?

The worst was brought on by my trying to control something I could not control. My wife, Pat, has a mental illness, and I kept trying to make sense of it. I wanted to save her from the pain. I wanted to save myself from the pain, too...

I had a period where I had what they call Major Depression. I hit a bump! I went into some pretty thorough therapy, and I have been ok since that time—sad sometimes, but nothing like before.

I remained able to work, and have a life, and I didn't have to take medicine...

I want to hear your story. For each of us has a different one... What makes you unique among others? What makes you the same as others?

What makes me the same is I have the same emotions, and feelings as anyone else.

What makes me unique is that God has graced me with certain talents that maybe not very many people have. Being an engineer is tough, and out of the populous as a whole. Not many people can do this job.

Another thing unique, is that I got to retire at age 52! People usually retire at 62, 57, or 55. I am so thankful!

How do you feel about where you are today? What makes you happy? What makes you sad?

I worked my butt off for so long! I had to worry about so many things that I don't have to worry about today.

I am quite happy about not needing to get up at a certain time. I can take as much time as I want at anything I want. I am in a good place today, and I am a grateful free spirit!

I'm looking for a T-shirt that says, "I don't want to! I don't have to! You can't make me! I'm retired!" That says it all!

What makes me sad is fighting! No matter which one of us starts it, it makes all the things I love mean nothing to me...

Do you have any regrets? If so, what are they?

I have very few regrets. I have some regrets that are unclear. I guess I regret the way I did certain things. I can't think of an example right now...

Maybe I regret our first camping trip, where we laid down next to a big rock. I regret freezing, in the name of sleeping under the stars! It's called youth...

What material thing really sings to you?

Things that I enjoy sing to me. Some people have material things, just to have material things. When I have something, I use it, and I enjoy it thoroughly!

If I don't think I'll like something, I don't buy it... I like things that work the way they're designed, and that are convenient.

If they don't work, I return them, or get a part from the company, and fix it.

What are 2 interests you have?

I have a whole list of interests! Go read it! (ha! ha!)

I love to camp, travel, work in my yard, fish, read, watch TV, and many, many more...

What would you say to God, if He was right in front of you?

I'd say thank you! Thank you for everything I have... My wife says God would say, "Well done, good and faithful servant"...

How long have you been afflicted with a mental illness?

Well, let's see, it started in my late teens all the way up through my early forties. It's been twenty some years...

What makes your life worth living?

It varies from day to day. Having a project in mind helps me get up in the morning, and gives me a purpose. Going to see something I've never seen before gives me a purpose— like the world's largest ball of twine, or the biggest frying pan, or the huge cross down in Texas.

Where would you be without mental health support?

I would be dead.

If you could tell the world your greatest 'dream', what would it be?

I would like everyone to be healthy, and get enjoyment from whatever they choose to do...

Summary:

I must say that my husband is about as normal a person as you will find. Normal isn't even in my vocabulary!

I have known him for 30 years, and through this interview I can say that he is a man of simple pleasures. I use to think he had expensive tastes...

He is still a stranger, after all this time we've been together.

All I know is, "He is love"... Isn't that enough to last an eternity?

Patricia A. Fisher

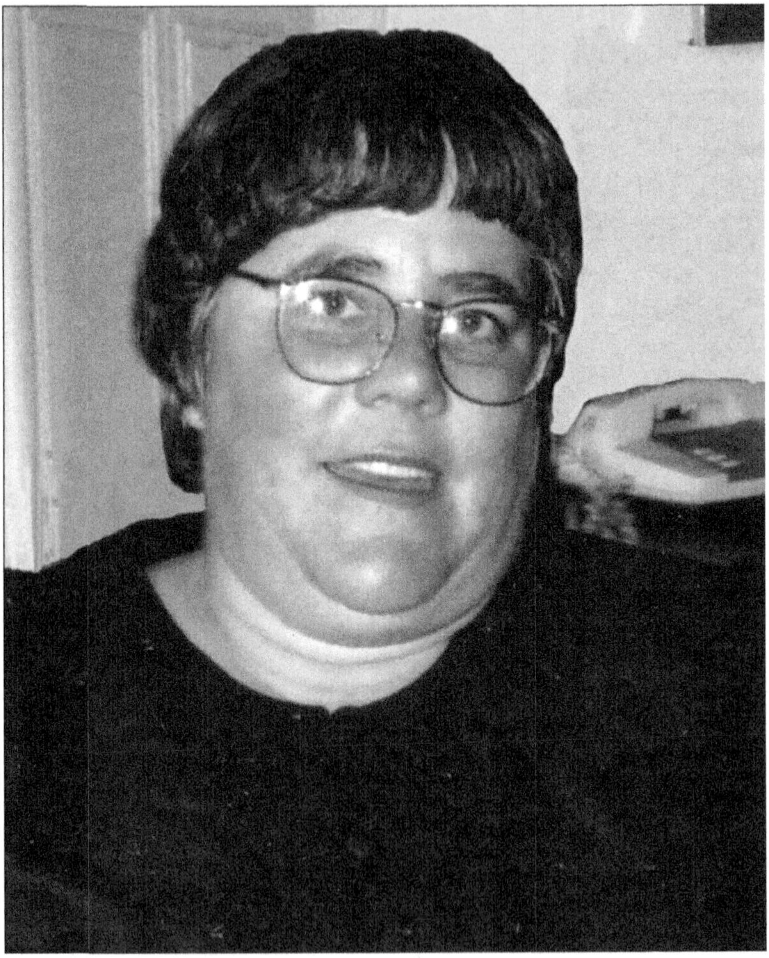

Patricia D. Wilson
What Is Your Story?

What are 3 things that keep you going while you are in the pits?

I have Jehovah God. He's my strength and my shield and my stronghold. I have my spiritual family. I have very loving support from my technician, Patti, at the Community Living Program, (CLP). She's worked long and hard with me for four years.

I'm sure there were times, when she wanted to pull her hair out at the roots thinking, "When is Patty ever going to get this?" She always hung in there with me.

She traveled with me through my many, many journeys, and I'd really like to say, "Thank you very much, Patti, for all the things you did for me. You are really going to be missed by me."

Now, when I'm home, I try to practice my skills, living in the moment, using my wise mind, realizing there are pros and cons to life.

If people choose not to understand I'm mentally ill, they have a problem, not me... I don't live a mental illness. I am a whole person!

There's just a part of you that has a mental illness?

Yes!"

What are 3 things you do to stay out of the pits?

I love being in the moment. I love being active in the community. I love helping people, and sharing scriptures with them, from Jehovah God's word. Patricia Fisher and I are sitting down here talking. I find that to be very comforting and soothing.

It shows to me that Patty Fisher cares. I like helping other people, like Patricia Fisher, who care in that capacity.

I was in the community helping an older lady, in the same way, and this really keeps me going. It helps me mentally, physically, and emotionally, and that keeps me from going into the pits!

You don't appear to be afraid of reaching out to help people or to ask for something—or any of those things.

No, I don't, because I really believe I have been commissioned by Jehovah God, to do just that very work.

My ministry is to reach out to others to give them that comforting message from the bible, and to even help them in personal ways in their lives. That makes me feel needed.
That's all I've ever wanted, all my life. I am now 48. I still want to feel needed, and I do feel needed when I reach out to others.

Tell me something about your past -- anything that comes to your mind.

I enjoyed the many vacations and travels I had the pleasure of taking, when I was in Europe with my parents and my brother.

We traveled extensively through Austria, Switzerland, Italy, and Oberamaga in western Germany.

I swam to the middle of the Hinter Sea, and back again. I had a race with my Mom and I won!

It was simply breathtaking to see, as a child, how so many people could get along in those towns, how we could converse—even with my limited German.

I thought it was really awesome being able to take in that fresh air, talking to people, eating the many fine foods and delicacies they prepared. Not many children have that opportunity.

What happened to bring on your affliction?

I was actually born with all my mental illnesses. I was born an alcoholic syndrome baby. My parents drank alcohol and still drink to this day...

When I was at the age of 8, I vividly recall, "My Dad came home drunk, went into the bathroom and passed out." Before he passed out, he said, "Hon, get my daughter out of here." I said to my Mother, "I know my Dad's drunk."

It was from birth that I had all these mental afflictions, and it was hereditary. There are many babies born today with mental illnesses.

Dr. Susan, of University Hospital, out on 9th and Colorado, said she was surprised that I did not have a "Drinking Gene". She said she was surprised I was not an alcoholic... I don't even keep alcohol in my house!

I want to hear your story. For each of us has a different one... What makes you unique among others? What makes you the same as others?

I realize that I have these illnesses, and that I am not 'an illness'. I am still a whole person, and capable of functioning with Jehovah God's help, and the professionals that work with me at CLP.

How do you feel about where you are today? What makes you happy? What makes you sad?

Well, I'm very happy I have Jehovah God in my life, my spiritual family, people like you in my life, and my family. They're all good support systems.

Jehovah God knows that, and once again I'm reiterating. I like to be very active out in the community to feel needed once again... **It makes you happy?**

Yes, it does, very happy! Jehovah God is a happy God, and He wants his people to be happy! **Are you ever sad?**

Again, I think of the many, many blessings Jehovah God has bestowed upon me.

**Do you have any regrets?
If so, what are they?**

No, I can't say that I have any regrets. Patricia, I'm happy where my life is right now, because I have Jehovah God, my spiritual family, my friends, and my family.

I don't have any regrets, because true Christians don't hold grudges. They lovingly forgive one another.

What material thing really sings to you?

I have my beautiful pure bred Tiger Cat. She's black with beige stripes.

She was another blessing bestowed upon me by Jehovah God three years ago. She came to me when she was one year old, from a beautiful pet shop! She's been a blessing to me ever since, a true blessing. Her name is Mickey Diana. **So she sings to you, huh?**

Oh Yeah!

Well, last night I was listening to our congregation book study on the phone. I was too sick to go. So my friends didn't pick me up, and she has a way of purring every time the congregation sings.

She sat there and listened to that entire two-hour meeting! **You're kidding!**

No, that's awesome... I have one cat. She's beautiful!

What are 2 interests you have?

I love going out into the community, talking with people about Jehovah God's word.
I also love doing that at Super Kmart, and at the same token, catching the good sales at Super Kmart!

What would you say to God, if He was right in front of you?

I want to thank you, Jehovah God, for each and every thing you have done for me, and that you are still doing for me, and everything that you are going to do for me, and for all the wonderful blessings.

How long have you been afflicted with a mental illness?

From birth.

What makes your life worth living?

Not only do I have Jehovah God in my life, but I have his Son, Jesus Christ.

He makes me see that it's awesome to continue living life just as it is... and he's not going to allow me to bare more than I'm capable of baring.

Where would you be without mental health support?

Where would I be without Jehovah God, and mental health support? I would still be in and out of the hospital.

Doctor Susan, when I was seeing her as a patient, said, "Patty, a lot of my patients are still in and out of the hospital. How do you do it?

I said, "I have Jehovah God in my life. He helps me!"

If you could tell the world your greatest 'dream', what would it be?

Living life in a peaceful new world, free of sickness and pain, where we're all well again, and that will be soon a reality—not a mere dream, but a reality...

Summary:

First of all, Patty would like to be referred to as a patient—not a client. To her the word client is very cold and damp. She says it is like a person going to a law office, or to a bank, or to an insurance company.

Patty says a patient is someone out to seek medical help, because they are ill, and they know that they are ill. She is emphatic, when she announces, "Please refer to me, Patty Wilson, as a patient!"

How can anyone sum up Patricia D. Wilson in a word, or a lot of words?

She is a believer who lives her life, first and foremost, as a woman on a mission. She had a rough start, but did not let her beginnings cause her to stop believing, or to stop sharing her love and energy.

She is a woman with a huge dose of courage! I admire her open devotion to her Jehovah God, and I understand a bit about her relationship to her higher power. For I have recently found mine...

I share her exuberance, when she speaks of the wonderful peace of forgiving...

It is such a waste carrying around resentment, anger, hate, and rage.

They rob us of our right to just be. They cause us to keep people away, because of mistrust. They are the culprits that make us throw people out of our hearts, instead of giving them the forgiveness they deserve.

They keep us from forgiving ourselves. For we, ourselves, are just human, too...

Yes, Patty Wilson brings about a soul searching in the most hardened individuals.

She is in touch with a power, so great, that it bubbles over onto you, and you get transformed.

Her love comes through her from her Jehovah God. She is truly an instrument of His peace, truth, and goodness. She is genuinely happy. Her Jehovah God wants it that way.

I am in awe of her energy, which comes from Him. I have never heard her complain, although she reports certain difficulties.

She is a walking dynamo, and she promotes a life of human kindness, as she moves through our communities and our world...

A world without Patty would be a bit less grateful and a bit less cheerful.

Our lives would be lacking one of God's own messengers.

Yes, I believe in the lessons I've learned, by letting this believer of goodness into my life.

Thank you, Patty, for sharing your truth...

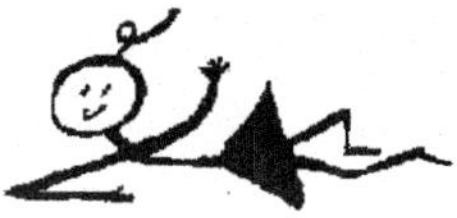

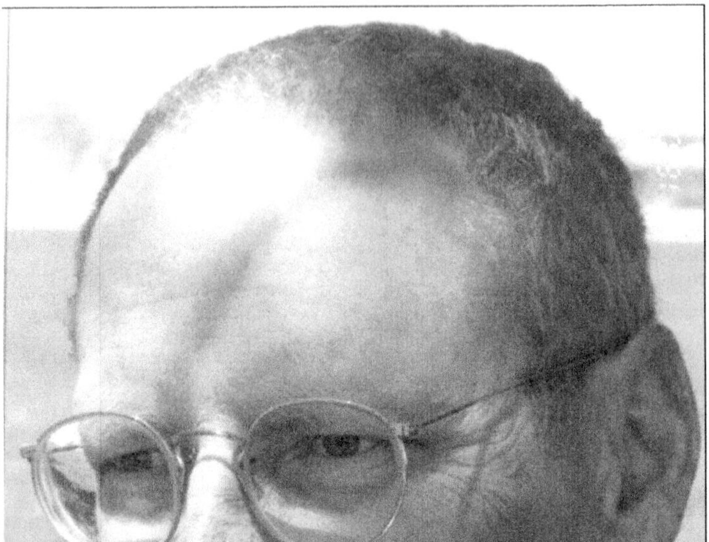

Chris "Nemo" Montgomery
What Is Your Story?

What are 3 things that keep you going while you are in the pits?

When I get in the pits, I feel that things will get better in the near future.

Also, I pretty well keep myself surrounded by good, supportive people. There are 6 or 7 of us. This is a big help.

I go to the gym, and it gives me someplace to go, as well as, it makes me feel good!

I hurt my hip, so I have to cut back on the treadmill. It should be ok soon.

And, last but not least, my photography and writing keeps me out of the pits, and gives me enjoyment.

This was my way of earning a living as a free lance writer and photographer. I traveled for many years, in my camper. I would stay in the desert for weeks -- all alone... I loved it!

What are 3 things you do to stay out of the pits?

Well, I am going to do an article for a news letter called "We Can".

The letter comes out quarterly, and my column is called, "Profiles in Recovery". This keeps me professional, which keeps me out of the pits. I just feel better!

"We Can" is an advocacy organization for mental health. I'm working for them on a volunteer basis.

Tell me something about your past -- anything that comes to your mind.

From age 15 to 18 I was heavily into drugs. I left home and became the traveler I speak about.

In my early twenties I lived in San Francisco, where I really grew up.

I've been in 17 countries. I began my adventures in the nineties writing travel pieces as I went from place to place in my camper.

What happened to bring on your affliction?

In 1997 I was diagnosed with Bipolar II, in 2000 with Borderline Personality Disorder, Post Traumatic Stress Disorder, and Generalized Anxiety Disorder.

I am now on S.S.D.I. as of this year. I'm not able to work.

Yet, I am going to enjoy my volunteer work, as it is very much like my career of writing and being a photographer.

I currently see a therapist, and I take the meds I am prescribed.

Also, I have never been married. Nor did I have children. I just never had that calling in life at all.

I want to hear your story. For each of us has a different one... What makes you unique among others? What makes you the same as others?

Umm, I didn't know interviews could be this tough! **spoken by a man who has interviewed hundreds!**

I don't know if this makes me unique, but I am kind of an intellectual, and a freethinker.

In my mid twenties, after I returned from Europe, I 'hit the skids'—literally! I went on skid row with an alcohol problem. I sobered up when I was age 32. I am 49 now...

The addictions sort of masked the mental health aspects. It's the same for a lot of people...

I seem to be delusional, at times. I met a young woman, who really understands how there can be a whole separate reality, while I'm living in another.

When I get like that, I call her, and we do a reality check.

How do you feel about where you are today? What makes you happy? What makes you sad?

What makes me happy, is being around supportive people. My traveling days are behind me now, and this is all a new life.

I am happy when I connect with new people, **pointing to us,** and when I'm doing other things that are just as worthwhile.

I'm sad whenever there's unresolved conflict between me and other people.
I have been a loner all my life, living in the desert. Now I'm trying to adjust to a life of being around people.

Do you have any regrets?
If so, what are they?

No, absolutely I don't! I'm not that kind of person with life.

As a matter of fact, I'll tell you something... If I was on my death bed right today, and someone came up to me and asked, "What didn't you do in life that you wish you would have done?" I would say, "nothing"!

I've done everything I ever wanted to do. And, now, I have no passion. I went to Egypt, and all over Europe.

There's absolutely nothing I'm dying to do...

I've lived my life thoroughly. I don't regret even the drugs, or alcohol. It was all part of the path.

What material thing really sings to you?

The desert was always my passion through life. It's kind of changed now. I'm not into going out there anymore. But that's what it was throughout my life...

It was my spirituality, too. I use to go out there and romp around. I was like a ten year old kid in a candy store! It's just unmatched beauty, and it's healing.

When asked about the perils of desert living, i.e. venomous creatures, I left them alone. They left me alone.

What are 2 interests you have?

1. Writing
2. Photography

What would you say to God, if He was right in front of you?

I don't even necessarily believe in God.

How long have you been afflicted with a mental illness?

I would say since age 16. That's when I saw my first mental health professional. It would be 33 years now, since I was diagnosed with Major Depression.

What makes your life worth living?

I think that it would be the core group of people that stay around me, care about me, and love me.

Also, I keep in my mind that the best is yet to come!

It's my hope that I will find somebody, and I won't have to be alone the rest of my life.

I can't believe I said that!

Where would you be without mental health support?

Boy, I shudder to think of that! I'm very, very fortunate that I have had the same therapist for three years.

Before that, I was in public health systems, being bumped and shuffled along from one intern to another—sometimes after only six months!

I'm also on a grant, which gives me a low fee. I know people who don't have this kind of opportunity.

Yes, I'm in a real fortunate position, but that could change quickly! I am worried about it a little bit.

I'm also in a good place, when it comes to medications. For I utilize the Prescription Assistance Programs (PAPS).

I am concerned about the budget cuts. They may shut down Fort Logan. Some of us, the more severe cases, would perhaps end up in prison. We wouldn't get the mental health services we need. We would be chastised, and treated like criminals! Some of us will go to Pueblo—where there won't be enough beds.

Some of us will be released into the community without adequate treatment.

The drop-in centers will be overwhelmed, and won't be able to handle the load.

The mental health systems won't get enough money to properly support us in our treatment.

If you could tell the world your greatest 'dream', what would it be?

I don't have any dreams. I've done everything I ever dreamed of. I've lived every dream that ever crossed my mind.

I'm incredibly fortunate. So, when I say I don't have any dreams, I'm being totally honest.

Having been a loner all my life, and rambling the world, even living in "flop houses", and doing everything I did— tells you what an adventurer I am.

I was always an explorer! I went to other countries just to see what made other cultures tick! I'm very multi-cultural.

But that's behind me now. I'm pushing 50. So comfort, and taking care of myself, are the precedents right now—especially with my mental health diagnoses in recent years.

Taking care of myself, and the insurance, and all those things are my priorities.

I'm not getting around to see the world anymore. Been there. Done that.

I'll tell you what comes up at this point. It's having a lady in my life—a significant other. **Well that would be a dream.**

Yes, I guess it is...

Summary:

Chris "Nemo" Montgomery is an unusual human being. He speaks from a place of 'knowing'.

He's a bit reserved, and intellectually inclined. Yet, his thinking is so like mine, that I kept saying, "Wow, that's just like me!"

It was so much fun listening to him, as he spoke his truth with our 'different' similarities.

"Nemo", is what he wants to be called.

The name, "Nemo", has a story behind it. Our "Nemo" is "Nemo-II". "Nemo-I" was named Everett Ruess.

In the 1930s, Ruess, a writer, artist, and nomad legend, traveled the desert with a horse and burro. He disappeared without a trace...

In the 1990s, "Nemo-II" traveled the same desert, as a writer and photographer.

Instead of a horse and burro, he had the luxury of a camper and motor cycle.

He is a professional man, with talent and initiative. This is important, when he goes out of his comfortable apartment, to interview & photograph other people— **Which he does very well.**

"Nemo" is just another one of those miracles, and he might not even know it!

He is a very interesting person, yet, similar to the rest of us. For his only wish left is to love and be loved.

Chris "Nemo" Montgomery, I know you'll find your dream...

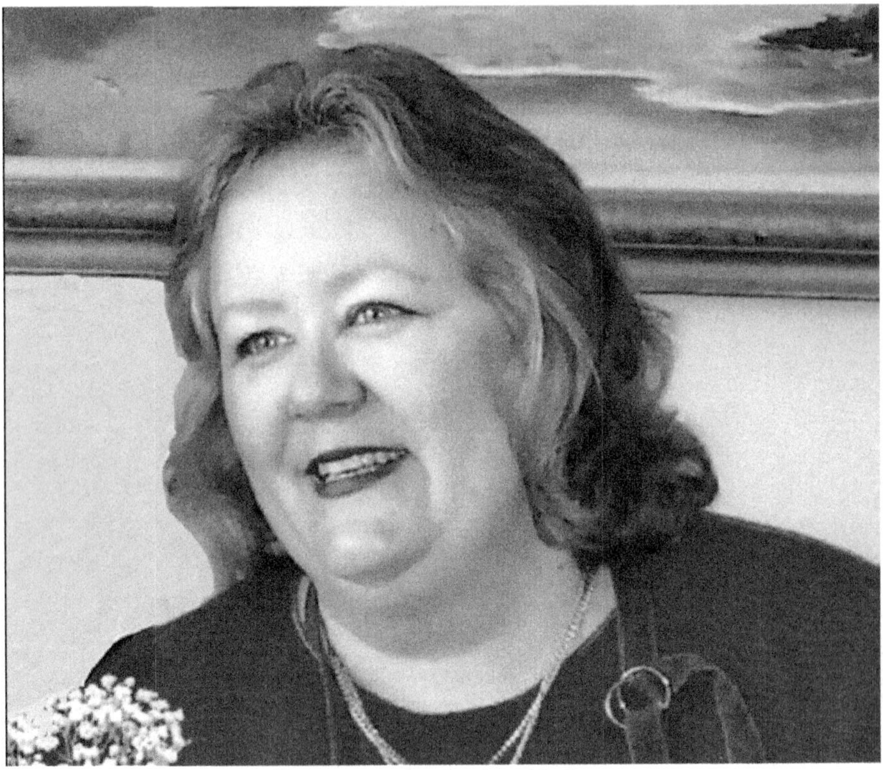

From a photo by Kate

Patricia A. Fisher
What Is Your Story?

What are 3 things that keep you going while you are in the pits?

When I go 'there', I usually lose my physical strength too.

So I cover myself up in bed, for a power rest, or just to feel secure. The next step is, when my husband comes in, and we talk a bit. This seems to get me to a place where I can call a mental health professional, or do one of My 25 Tools for Living. **I printed them in my book, "From This Day Forward".**

By the time I do all of this, I am ready to do something like make dinner, watch TV, etcetera.

What are 3 things you do to stay out of the pits?

These days I am real busy with my writing, and my business, "ITSMEEE" Industries. Writing a book, and publishing it, is very much like having a baby.

You have it under your wing for awhile. Then you've done all you can do, and it goes into someone else's hands.

I've wondered why I am still alive. Then, I realized that I have this spark in me that keeps me going...

When I am suicidal, or just feeling down, I never can take my life. It's that spark...

I'm finding I have some interests I never internalized--reading, TV, camping, traveling, and being with my husband, or our friends.

Tell me something about your past-- anything that comes to your mind.

Umm, I choose to comment on the positive. Anyone in my past is forgiven. I can go back to where I lived growing up, and it no longer hurts. The stuff I did causes me no pain.

Could 35 years of therapy have anything to do with this?

One day I said to my husband, "I forgave my parents!" It just happened!

I started forgiving myself, and everybody else! What a gift and what a relief...

My family is also in the category of human beings. What a concept! I forgive all humans—including myself. This makes me smile with my heart.

What happened to bring on your affliction?

It started, I believe, when Mom took us away, in the middle of the night. Daddy was at work. Can you imagine how he felt, when he entered the house?

I feel that, in the sixth grade, I started getting ridged. This is where my guidance stopped...

Lack of guidance was major in my 'creation' of 'Super Humans'...

Then I went to New York, and a lot of people know what that's like. New York can either make you or break you. I guess I let it break me... I ended up in Kings County Hospital, and I was there 3 months. This was the beginning of my affliction.

I'd rather not discuss that anymore...

I want to hear your story. For each of us has a different one... What makes you unique among others? What makes you the same as others?

I'm unique, because there's nobody like me! **Giggle Giggle.**

I write from my soul. God seems to be in charge of what I write now days. It's as if He comes right through my pen.

I'm unique, because I have a calling to be an author, as I practice loving people...

I am similar to others. I fall down, and get right back up again!

I don't know if many folks would call themselves a warrior, like I do.

My resilience is probably common. I tend to believe that everyone has a warrior-like way of facing their demons (some more than others).

What makes me happy, and a bit unique, is my awareness that zillions of people are living a life of service. They care so much, they want to contribute.

How do you feel about where you are today?
What makes you happy?
What makes you sad?

Today, my business is becoming slightly lucrative. I love to see a purchase order! I love to talk business!

Before, I would cry if a form was sent to me. I didn't understand the 'lingo'.

These days, I fill them out, and sometimes enjoy it. This makes me happy, too.

My sadness is very rare these days. I get slightly melancholy, when I think about my Mom passing away. I miss those 2-hour talks we had...

It has been over a year...

**Do you have any regrets?
If so, what are they?**

We worked in our respective ways for 30 years.

Both of us contributed to our marriage, to our finances, and even had fun once in awhile! Quaint idea huh?

I have been treated with caring, respect, and truth, by 'my' Dennis and my mental health professionals.

My only regret is, when Mom had a heart attack, on September 11th, we weren't thinking well, and did not help her cross the street until she said something.

She had that heart attack while making a pie in her own home.

What material thing really sings to you?

I love pajamas, pretty dresses, jeans, and my black outfits!

I love my little red, V.W. Beetle! It came to me as a retirement present. I waited a long time and I am thankful.

I have plenty that sings to me, wooden spoons, rolling pins, Leather chairs, sunshine, and spring.

What are 2 interests you have?

I like writing books and talking with interesting people.

What would you say to God, if He was right in front of you?

I'd say, "Good morning God", not "Good God it's morning!"

This would, at least, be a good beginning...

How long have you been afflicted with a mental illness?

About 35 years.

What makes your life worth living?

Caring, Respect and Truth
My new found faith,
My marriage,
And unconditional love.

Where would you be without mental health support?

I would be dead, most likely. I was into drugs back then, and not taking care of myself. This lead me toward an almost certain demise.

If you could tell the world your greatest 'dream', what would it be?

I would like for every person to have more happiness, more fun, some peace of mind and at least one person to love.

Summary:

The late Dee Stanley told Pat that her book, "ITSMEEE" On My Journey Home", showed that she had gone from the darkness to the light. Thanks (angel) Dee.

Pat is unique in that she has a great mental health problem that has persisted for 35 years. However, with therapy and the proper medications, she has developed 25 tools that she uses to get through life.

Mental health professionals, treating her with caring, respect, and truth, have helped her to achieve the remarkable.

She has written from her heart and soul, and with God's help, developed this into 9 books.

She practices sharing and caring every day. She tries very hard to put into action, caring, respect, and truth, for everyone she has contact with.

Love is her middle name.

Summary and Interview
By D. H. Fisher

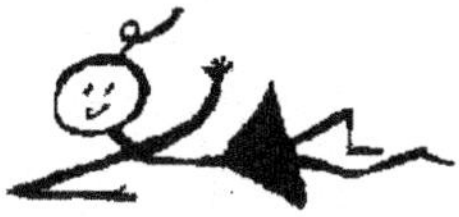

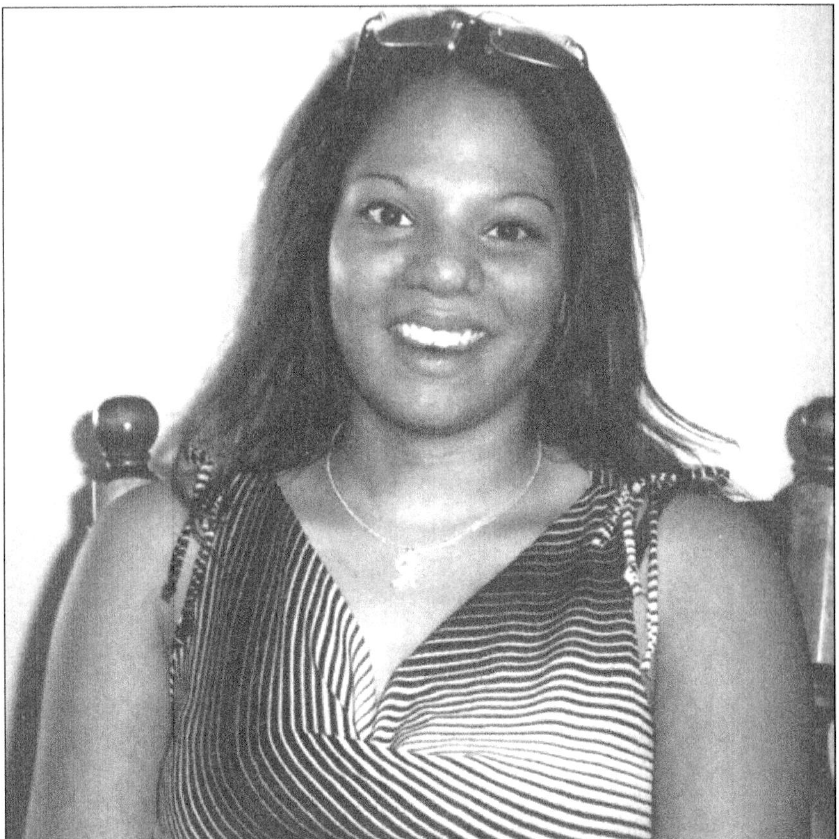

Rachel Vogel
What Is Your Story?

What are 3 things that keep you going while you are in the pits?

Praying
Listening to music
Talking to my Mom

What are 3 things you do to stay out of the pits?

Pray
Write down my problems
Take it day by day

Tell me something about your past -- anything that comes to your mind.

I was 17, when I was diagnosed with Bi-Polar...

What happened to bring on your affliction?

My friend and me were talking, and I diagnosed myself! Then I went to a Psychiatrist, and he said I was Bi-Polar. Then I was put on medicine.

I'm not on it now. I'm fine! I might have my days, but it's not bad.

The medication I'm on makes me heavy, and I don't want to be on that right now.

I want to hear your story. For each of us has a different one...

What makes you unique? What makes you the same? I was raised by a single Mother (off of welfare). I'm mixed. I do not know my biographical Father. I'm the only one out of 6 cousins who has Bi-Polar. I have, probably 10 or 12 half brothers and sisters from my Father (that I do not know).

Um, I do not know what else. **Your teeth are beautiful.**

Thanks. I got em from my Mom. **Rachel and I chuckle...**

Mmmmm. Mistakes Some—everything makes me the same as others, but, in some ways, I'm unique and different.

Well, I mean, I am human. I do error. I look the same as anyone else. **We laugh.** Well not really... I have eyes, teeth and a nose. I can't compare myself to other people, 'cause I have a different way of seeing things—as most people. So, I can't categorize me as just a plain Jane girl.

How do you feel about where you are today?
What makes you happy?
What makes you sad?

Um, I got myself a job, but I got laid off the week before Christmas.

I'm doing alright, I mean, I'm going to find a job, I mean, Today I'm doing good! I have people around me who love me. I have my own apartment and car. My bills are paid. So, I'm alright.

What makes me happy is being around my close friends, just hangin' out, going out shopping, reading, and everything!

What makes me sad is ignorant people. That's just people who don't understand me (who think I'm wrong).

Um, racism and violence today, just little things, just everything...

September 11th, and all that stuff. The world is coming to an end. It's just kind of sad. The world's kind of falling, slowly...

Do you have any regrets? If so, what are they?

My regrets are being too trustworthy with people, and telling people about my sickness, and then they throw it back in my face.

Just being too trustworthy--I'm too open with people and I regret that, 'cause it comes back and hurts me, so... And that's it!

What material thing really sings to you?

My cell phone sings to me, literally! **another chuckle**

What are 2 interests you have?

Finishing college
Becoming a singer
(I haven't even started...)
It sounds like a wonderful plan!

What would you say to God, if He was right in front of you?

Thank you for making me who I am, and forgiving me for all the wrong I've done, and for never forsaking me. That's what I'd say to him.

How long have you been afflicted with a mental illness?

(All my life) I just was diagnosed with it at 17. I mean, I've had it since I was a baby. My Mom was waiting for me to come to terms with it myself, I think. 'Cause there was always something wrong, but they just couldn't pin point it.

I finally pin pointed it, so that it all made sense.

I'm very mild, I mean, with everything I've gone through, I should be down in the dumps. I'm not. I'm only on 5 milligrams of Ziprexa. So I'm not that mild, but I can become it.

What makes your life worth living?

Knowing I can get out of this, and make myself better. It's like a purpose, yah.

I tried to commit suicide, and it didn't work.

Obviously, God has a plan for me. So, there's no point in trying to do it again. You know, just taking it day by day.

Where would you be without mental health support?

Dead.

Finding out I have a mental problem, and that I wasn't crazy, made sense to me. I could fix it. I'm always gonna be Bi-Polar, but I can be on medication to fix that.

I don't want people to look down on me for it, like my Mom and my best friends. One of my best friends is Bi-Polar, too, and we interact.

If you could tell the world your greatest 'dream', what would it be?

To be on stage, at Madison Square Garden, with 20,000, people, singing a song I wrote, back to me... That's my highest dream.

Well, Rachel, I wish I had more questions! It's been just delightful!

Summary:

Rachel is a beautiful, and interesting, young woman. She told her truth in such a way, that I got goose bumps!

I would be thrilled, if a lot of young people, had aspirations and dreams for their future like Rachel has.

Rachel feels she can reach the sky, and it makes my heart sing. For we all have a chance to contribute something meaningful.

Rachel has come a very long way, on a hard rocky road. I feel that she has found her higher power, and they have an amazing connection!

Be careful walking too close to her. She could ignite you to your soul, and you might begin to dream your dreams, and attain them also...

She has people around her who love her. She has interests.

Her intelligence comes through the answers she gives, which told me she has thought about life.

I found her to be ageless, which I have seen in other people, from time to time. To me it means she has a depth beyond her years, and she appears to be ready for her young life to unfold.

I want to be there, at Madison Square Garden, when we all sing with our heart and soul, a lovely song by Rachel. I'll be the first person to stand and applaud her work. That is, if her Mom isn't there. If she is, I may just have to be second!

Rachel speaks of talking with her Mom. She explains that it is one of her necessary things to do.

What a wise choice, to spend lots of time with your Mom! It is preparation for the day, you begin to see clearly, that Mom was really smart after all...

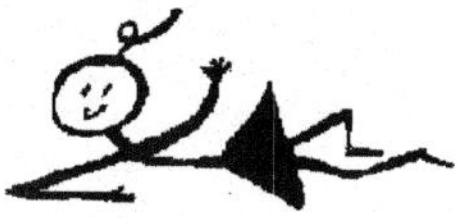

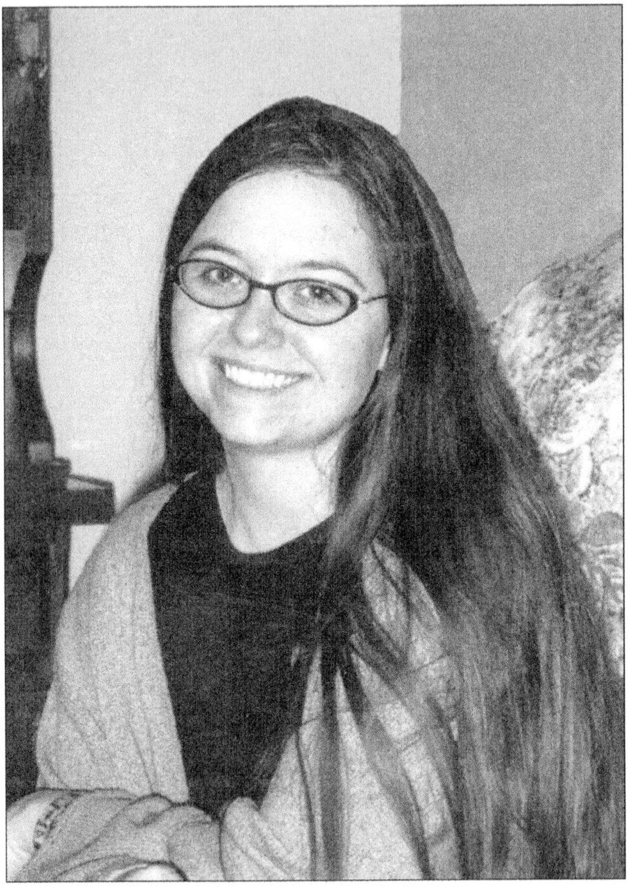

Jennifer Harbin
What is Your Story?

What are 3 things that keep you going while you are in the pits?

I use to have this magnet hanging on my refrigerator that says, "This too shall pass".

Knowing the bigger picture, and remembering from past experience, that I'll come out of it. My moods go like the tides. Sometimes I'm depressed, and sometimes I'm not...

I have a good support system. I have a few people in my life who are very understanding and compassionate. I can talk to them about anything I need to. They're nonjudgmental and that helps a lot.

A third thing—remembering how I've been in the past—just remembering the positive times in my life, and know that they will return. Just being positive to the best of my ability...

My bi-polar group is a big part of my life! I love to go there every week!

What are 3 things you do to stay out of the pits?

Keep moving. Keep going. I don't mean moving like my physical body. I don't get stuck in a rut thinking how crumby I feel.

I try to notice when I'm isolating myself. I get out of the house—call some friends… I go for a walk in the city park, and look at the geese and ducks. Um, just engaging with other people seems to help a lot.

I take my medicine every day. I'm very good at that! I set my alarm for 9am, 4pm and 9pm, and it goes off. I immediately go take my medicine…

If I keep it at those intervals, it seems to help me be more steady. If I don't take my medicine in an hour, I will be crying. My self esteem will have hit rock bottom. I'll be paranoid, and it's just an awful experience!

Tell me something about your past—anything that comes to your mind.

Anything, huh? **We chuckle.**

When I was 14 or 15, that's when I started getting depressed, but I didn't tell anybody.

My dad also bought me my first camera that year, and I learned how to use the camera. I tried it out on our trip to Europe, and I ruined all the pictures! I didn't want to read the instructions. I just wanted to figure it out myself. I ruined a lot of pictures...

Then I decided to go to school (college) to learn how to use the camera. I love taking pictures, and they're not half bad... I love exhibiting them in coffee shops or contests. I still have my old camera ...

I found out, that using my camera, was a good way to get out of my head, and into the outside world.

When I stay inside my head, I just drive myself crazy. I just get worse and worse. So, using my camera was a great outlet for being productive, and 'out-of-here', out of my head...

What happened to bring on your affliction?

My affliction... hmm... I kind of trace it really far back, when I was adopted. So one of the things I get stuck on is being abandoned. I think everybody feels that as well.

Umm... So I take relationships very personally! I really latch onto people—something I'm trying to learn to do better.

I had a series of people leaving in my life, and the depression started when I was 14 or 15. My first huge bout of depression was when I was visiting home, and my great grandmother had just died. It was a bad time—not very happy. I was sitting around the house, thinking about my granny.

The day before I left, my Mother started talking to me. She said she wanted to tell me how she really felt about me. Um... and she said some pretty cruel things that I can't believe she said to me.

She said that I had no mind of my own, can't think for myself, so far I'm a failure, haven't finished college, why I had not moved on, that I don't know what I want to do, and the list goes on and on.

I kind of pretended like it didn't hurt my feelings. Weeks after that I completely crashed, and had to be hospitalized. For several years I was depressed the whole time—except for this manic episode.

I was having trouble in a relationship. There was a guy who was not stalking me, but was very threatening, and it scared me to death!

So I left Colorado to live with my aunt and uncle in North Carolina. That's when my first manic episode started, because I started taking an antidepressant. It just brought it on really quick! I went very high...

I want to hear your story. For each of us has a different one... What makes you unique? What makes you the same?

I was adopted when I was 2 weeks old, to 2 wonderful parents. I grew up on a farm in Texas, where we had cows and horses, and chickens. Ummm... There was my Mom, my Dad, my brother and me.

My parents were very religious, and they provided a rigid structure, which was actually very helpful. Well, me, I like everything spelled out.

They had very high standards. I was a straight-A student from the moment I started school.

We moved to another part of Texas, when I was in 5th grade. From that moment on I became very active in school—student council, track and field, basketball, and all that kind of stuff.

I didn't like school very much.

I didn't have many friends. I wasn't in a group. I had friends, but I wasn't in a group.

Um… After I graduated, I decided to go to Belgium, as an exchange student. That went pretty well for a little bit, but that's when I started to have some pretty bad bouts with depression.

When I returned, and enrolled in the University of North Texas, I got on medication for the first time.

Then I moved to Colorado. I didn't want to be with my parents anymore. I wanted to get out of the house, so I started to go to school again.

I never received a degree. I get really depressed, when I go to school, so I haven't been able to finish that.

I think what makes me unique, is that I face my problems straight on—no messing around. When I started therapy, I just dove right in. For three years I was out of commission, because I was really dealing with some big issues.

Once I started educating myself, the scary stuff, which was the darkness, came out into the light. It didn't cause so much fear, and I could move forward.

Oh... I'm the same as anyone else.

I experience joy, sadness, happiness, anger. I have ambitions, I want to be loved, and have a feeling of completeness, just like anyone else...

How's that? **That was beautiful!**

How do you feel about where you are today?
What makes you happy?
What makes you sad?

I'm very pleased where I am today. The way I am today, is probably the best I've ever been! To come out of that deep depression, where I'd been for several years, feels good!

Now that I have medicine, I am more positive. I don't cry all the time. I can really relate to people. I am more sociable. I love it!

What makes me sad? I have to take medicine! I'm still dealing with that. I hate it!

Sometimes I hate it so much, I don't take it for several hours, and then I feel like crap! So I go take it. I'm still learning to deal with it... I wish I didn't have to take 9 different medications a day!

Something that makes me happy is, I like to be around people now. I love laughter.

I think, the essential thing in life, is to play and to laugh at yourself. I couldn't do that in the past. Boy is my life better, when I just laugh at myself for making a mistake.

I love being in nature, being around people, and taking walks, and just leading a down-to-earth life!

**Do you have any regrets?
If so what are they?**

In my whole entire life? I'll have to say, "No, I don't." I think everything that happened in my life happened for a reason.

I wouldn't be who I am, right now, if I regretted things, or didn't do things, or passed up opportunities. No, I don't think I do.

What material thing really sings to you?

You mean, speaks out to me, or what do you mean? **I mean, what makes you feel good?**

Little bitty things—I love teeny tiny things. I collect turtles, penguins, dolphins—anything tiny.

Right now, in my life, I'm more interested in experiences.

Like this past Thanksgiving and Christmas, my Mom taught me her recipes! That was pretty precious to me!

My cat is not a thing to own, but it's my friend. I like him a lot. He makes me pretty happy. **Well, don't tell him he's a material thing!**

No! **We laugh...** He's not a thing at all!

What are 2 interests you have?

You already know a few of them, actually.

Photography, little bitty things, playing—let's see... I love reading.

I'm really interested in criminology. I like to read true crime books. Those are pretty interesting. I like oil painting, and charcoals. I'm repeating myself, when I mention my walks in the park...

What would you say to God, if He were standing right in front of you?

That's a hard question, but I'll go with, "Thanks for never leaving me alone." I have pretty much had hope the whole time. Sometimes, in my darkest hour, I thought I was all alone, but I really wasn't. So, "Thank you for giving me hope."

How long have you been afflicted with a mental illness?

Depression since 14 or 15, but I was diagnosed with Bi-Polar a year and 2 months ago.

What makes your life worth living?

Well, I'll have to say, "for myself", my goal of taking care of myself, loving myself, and then being able to spread that love outside of me. I can't do that until I first learn to take care of me.

There are so many mysteries that are just around the corner, you know?

You never know when a beautiful miracle will come along. I don't know. I love surprises...

Where would you be without mental health support?

I would be dead. Um... had I not got help, I would be dead.

If you could tell the world your greatest 'dream', what would it be?

My greatest dream... I want to leave the world a bit better. There is a quote, by Ralph Waldo Emerson, about success.

I'd like to be a success according to that quote, and that's "to leave the world a little bit better, either by a garden patch, or a healthy child. To know that one life has breathed easier because of you, that is to have succeeded."

I would like to use every breath in my body to help myself, but to help others too.

Having a mental illness does not have to stop me...

Summary:

Well, Jennifer, your last sentence is quite powerful! Let's bottle it! We could make millions—no, billions...

As Jennifer and I were talking, I kept having that familiar feeling that I was speaking to a fellow warrior. She is not one to quit easy.

She uses her photography in much the same way that I use my writing. It helps her get outside herself and it is a valid contribution to the world.

She is wise. She harbors important things, like good friends, nature, and her medicine. She seems to have a way of managing her life very well, and she knows what she needs.

We shared laughter and warm conversation.

The time passed quickly, like it does when people are enjoying themselves. It was just one person sharing their life experience with another.

She spoke of "the darkness coming out into the light". Since this happened, she has been able to go forward with her life.

If we could bottle yet another piece of this interview, it would be the removal of inner darkness. For so much can be 'festering' where there is no light.

Thank you, Jennifer, for reminding us of the good that is in the world, and you have already made the world "a little bit better"...

Patricia A. Fisher

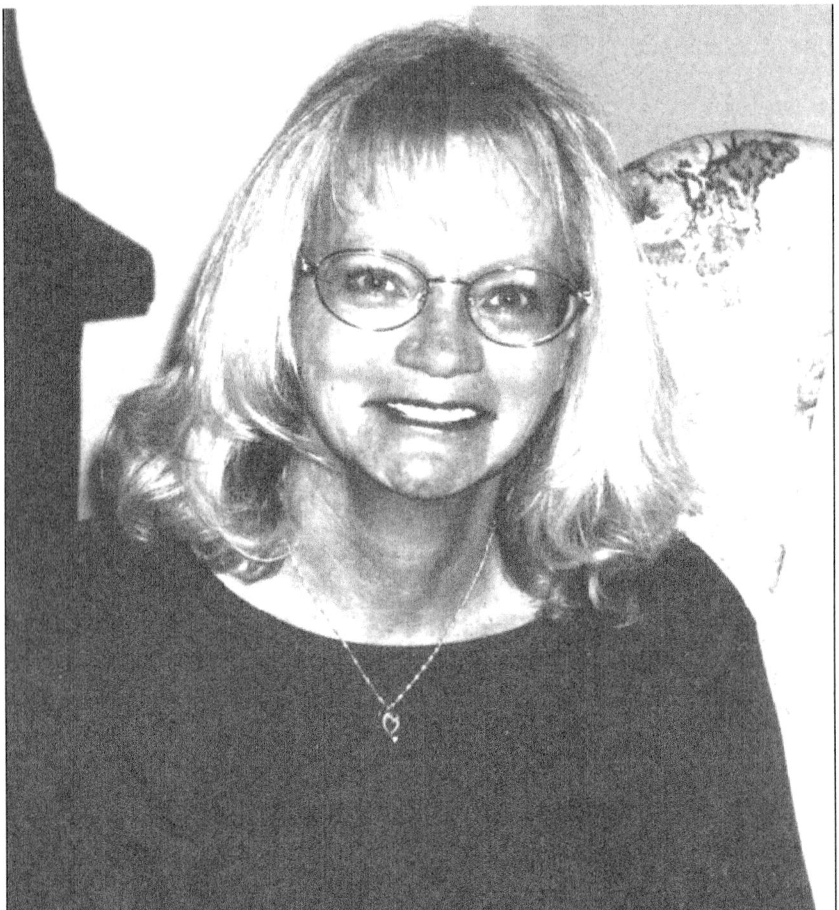

Marilyn Rogers
What Is Your Story?

What are three things that keep you going while you are in the pits?

I would say they are my daughter, my niece, and although my Mom has passed away, I would say, the memory of my Mom. She always wanted me to make it.

What are three things you do to stay out of the pits?

I do a lot of talking with my daughter. Uh, I try to do some painting. It calms me down so I can gather my thoughts.

I have a 16 year old niece who keeps me going. She just got a car, and all that fun stuff. She is in track.

So it's for them that I keep going.

I make it a point to talk to somebody, or go out for a walk. I do have 2 little Chihuahuas, that are my life. So, a lot of times, I'll just take them and go out for a walk.

Tell me something about your past—anything that comes to your mind.

It would probably be the birth of my daughter. That was the most exciting, most enjoyable, most precious moment in my life.

She was all I ever wanted. I wanted a blonde haired, tiny baby girl, and that's what I got! I got a blue-eyed blonde, and 4 lbs 9 oz, and she's been everything I wanted!

She's never done anything to disappoint me. In my low times, this girl has gone out, and literally bought food, and hand fed me. She's missed school to be there for me or my Mom. She's gone through a lot, and she just means the world to me...

I dedicated to her, "The First Time I Ever Saw Your Face" by Roberta Flack. I made an album of her life (my daughter) from birth, and put that on it. It's a beautiful song! I love it!

My daughter is not the apple of my eye. She's the whole tree! I would do anything for her, and her for me. She's my life.

What happened to bring on your affliction?

It's always been there. I have borderline personality (disorder), major depression, and P.T.S.D. (post traumatic stress disorder).

The borderline has been there since I was 13. The major thing that I would have to say, that really pushed me over the edge, was the death of my Mom...

That was in 95—December of 95. I lost my Dad and my Mom in that month. (my Dad in 1988 and my Mom in 1995)

My Mom and I were just as close as my daughter and I are. It was like we did everything together. **The Moms are the hardest to lose.**

Yah... She had C.O.P.D. for 6 years, so I had to take care of her 24-7, while trying to take care of two acres of land, my daughter, and jobs.

I was never 'spotted' by my family. I never got to go out to dinner, to movies... When it came time for my Mom to pass away, she passed away at home.

I was partially responsible for her death, because of giving her Morphine every 45 minutes. It was to ease the pain, and help her breathe, but it also hastened her death. I feel guilty in my heart...

I want to hear your story. For each of us has a different one... What makes you unique? What makes you the same?

Ok, I think maybe my ability to listen, um, I hear people.

I don't just listen, but I hear them! I'm very supportive. I go through a lot with some of my friends that I've met. A lot of times they put a lot on me, but I do the best I can to help them out.

I'm a mother hen. I like to take them under my wing. I think not everybody can do that.

I don't really get 'stung', but when I do, it's really a big one!

Just recently, I went through one with a friend. I had to pull away from her for 2 months. It was sending me into a depression where I would stay in bed for days.

I finally told her, "I love you. I care about you, but you just can't do this to me anymore." It's pretty much ended...

As far as your question, "What makes you the same", I'm only human... **That's powerful!**

How do you feel about where you are today? What makes you happy? What makes you sad?

Uh, on the good side, I'm happy to be out of the half-way homes. I'm a little bit sad, because I was a little bit too giving, and ended up losing my home. It was my inheritance.

It was due to some wrong choices I made with people. It makes me really sad!

I lost a lot, but I didn't lose everything. I still have my dignity, and I feel what I did was right.

What the kids did to me is on them, and they have to answer for it. I took some kids in off the street, to help them get jobs, and get back in school. They were 18 and 19. The girl was pregnant with a mixed child, and I did the best I could for them.

They took advantage of it. They ruined my car. They caused me to lose my house.

They wouldn't let me talk to my therapist. They would intercept the calls.

So, it really got to the point where it got very sad.

I look on it now, that I learned a lesson, and that I tried to help.

So, I'm glad to be out of the homes and stuff, but by the same token, I'm sad I had to sell the place I liked. I had to move on.

What makes me happy? There again, I have to go with my daughter!

She and I have unlimited long distance!

We're calling each other 2 and 3 times a day, just for chitchat.

It's marvelous, because neither of has to say, "Oh, we've been on the phone too long, or it's gonna cost me a ton!"

It's wonderful! I am just ecstatic about it! When I hear that special long distance ring I'm like, "My baby's on the phone!"

It just lifts me, because she understands. She is a child that was raised by a Mother who had borderline personality disorder. She didn't know when I was going to fly off the handle!

She was raised with this all her life, and she still stuck by me. That to me is just incredible, just incredible! She hangs in there, whether her Mom barks at her, or laughs at her.

I mean, it can be as simple as when she goes to put powdered sugar on a pancake. When the sugar fell, and hit the table, it went poof! She didn't know if I was going to laugh or bite her head off!

When I started laughing, she said she never heard me laugh so hard, but she was on pins and needles wondering how I was going to take it.

I have to give her a lot of credit for putting up with me.

It's a blessing. I love to talk to her!

She's 7 weeks pregnant. I'm like, finally! She's settled down, and she works hard, and she and her boyfriend are just like two peas in a pod... He treats her good. She treats him good, and the world just keeps on going!

What makes me sad is probably the early loss of my parents. My Dad was only 55, and my Mom was 62. So I felt kind of cheated. They were just wonderful parents. I just idolized them!

Sometimes, when I'm looking up at a sunset, I'll say, "Mom, you're missing this. This is one of your favorite times!"

My Dad would tell me of a good price at a gas station.

It makes me sad, but they have been gone so long, I feel I'm beginning to deal with it...

Do you have any regrets? If so, what are they?

I could say, taking in these kids, but I don't regret that, because we did have a good time before things got heated.

I took care of her new baby, who was born in June. So, on one hand, I kind of regret taking them in, but, on the other hand I feel I did the best I could.

I do regret my daughter having to grow up under a Mom 'that she doesn't know what she's going to do…' I wish I would have been diagnosed earlier. I knew there was something wrong, and I was afraid, if someone found out, I'd lose my daughter.

My daughter came home with a new word. Her teacher would teach them one every little while. She said, Mom that's what you are. (The word's meaning was "somebody who talks a lot!") **We laughed.**

I told her that, even on the back of my report card from kindergarten, the teacher wrote that I talked too much in class. So, I got the gift of gab!
We giggle...

What material thing really sings to you?

And don't say the radio!
I laugh and she doesn't...

She says, "The last professional picture I have of my Mom." Whenever I go into the hospital or the halfway houses, I take a picture of my Mom, and my daughter.

My friends would ask if they could call my Mother, "Mom". I'd say, "You can call her Mom, but she's mine!"

I look at her picture, and she sort of speaks to me—not in a bad way. She just says to me, "Hang in there baby!" It's just her smile and her warmth...

My Dad and my Grandma were always at each other, but when my Dad died, Grandma asked if she could be buried right next to him, so she could "give him heck all the way to heaven!" **I laugh loudly!**

Grandma idolized my Dad. So, when they passed, we buried my Mom on one side of my Dad, and my Grandma on the other!

Like Dennis and your Mom, those relationships don't come along every day...

What are two interests you have?

I love reading something true! It doesn't matter if it's a doctor, you know, who grew up in the ghetto and, becomes... It's called, "Healing Hands".

I love to read anything true—whether it's crime, law, whatever...

I was in Germany when my ex-husband was in the service.

To this day, I read books of holocaust survivors. My daughter had a class, where they brought in a husband and wife who had been in, I think, Auschwitz.

I was so excited! I said to my daughter, "Please ask if I can come too!" So I got to meet these people! They signed my book of "Schindler's List".

When I was in Germany, I went to one of the concentration camps.

My other passion would be the painting. Because I like to paint so much, I'm going to give my paintings to a nursing home.

I'll just tell them, "Put it in someone's room, who doesn't have family..."

What would you say to God, if He was right in front of you?

Oh Lord, I don't want to go there! Um, I saw a bumper sticker once that said, "Heaven won't have me, and hell is afraid I'm going to take over!" **We laugh again!**

Right now, I'm dealing with blaming God, being angry at God, and hating God, and anything else you can think of, because of taking my parents. God may not have taken them, but He allowed it.

Therefore, He made me an orphan, just to make me stand up and make me be me! But, what a way to do it! What a rotten way...

I struggle with it. I really do! I do believe in God, like a new born baby, that's a miracle! The developing of a baby, that's got to be instilled by God!

I just haven't been able to get over the anger and the hurt, and I hold Him responsible...

I know it's wrong, and I'm working on it. One of these days, He's going to say, "You're one of the worst cases I've seen yet! **Smile... I was going to give you one of my books, but I think you need all four!"**

We laughed again... We keep saying funny things, and laughter comes easy. I'm amazed at how strong my fellow mental health consumers are...

We discuss how we are survivors and warriors, she and I. We don't like it when people don't fight for themselves and their mental health.

What I would probably say to Him is, "Thanks for taking my Mom and Dad to heaven, and watching over them." They keep me going. They give me the strength to keep going...

I know my Mom and Dad would not want me to give up with suicide, or give up and walk the streets in oblivion. They're watching over me. I keep going for them.

How long have you been afflicted with your mental illness?

The borderline personality disorder started when I was about 13.

My depression started in about 1981, after my husband left.

What makes your life worth living?

I know what you're going to say! You do? Go ahead and tell me! **I don't tell her.**

It's my puppies, my grandbaby, my daughter. I love to help people out. Put me in a nursing home. Put me in a daycare center. I'd love it, because those are my favorites— the young and the old...

I don't have to worry if I love myself, because I get enough from others (like a big old smile from a child).

Where would you be without mental health support?

Dead. 'Cause, at times the depression got bad. With the borderline personality, you have the tendency to get so angry, that you cut.

I am a cutter. I haven't for quite awhile, but that was the only way I could bring myself back to reality. I was told, by a therapist, that the reason a borderline person will hurt themselves, with whatever they choose, is that it's their last step before suicide...

To cause themselves pain is to help them snap back to reality. It's like slapping somebody in the face, and saying, "Stop it!"

Without mental health help, suicide would have been very easy for me. Even if I hurt people, I needed to say to them, "If you love me, let me go...!"

I've just lately been able to cry. I'll cry and what a relief!

If you could tell the world your greatest 'dream', what would it be?

My biggest dream is for people to understand and realize that we're no different from anybody else. Um, just because I take meds, for mental illness, I'm no different than people who take them for anything!

I want people to wake up and quit putting the stigma on everybody!

My greatest dream is if people could accept people for who they are, and what they are.

Summary:

Well, how can I sum up an interview like this one? How can I define a person like Marilyn? There's no way, but I will share my thoughts with you.

I find that I did not portray all the humor that we enjoyed. We laughed at things that sometimes use to put us at hell's door.

We laughed at our similarities, and at the joy of just sharing with each other.

Marilyn shared her life's experience, with the innocence of a child. Her truth came through, as refreshing as a cool spring rain. Yet, it was filled with the depth of a humble human being.

It is a gift to be able to tell all, so that you can give love and maybe help someone else.

The person, we call Marilyn, came to me from far away. This is so, because I feel like I've known her a long, long time.

We appeared to know each other from one end of the continuum to the other. Our souls met like 2 old friends.

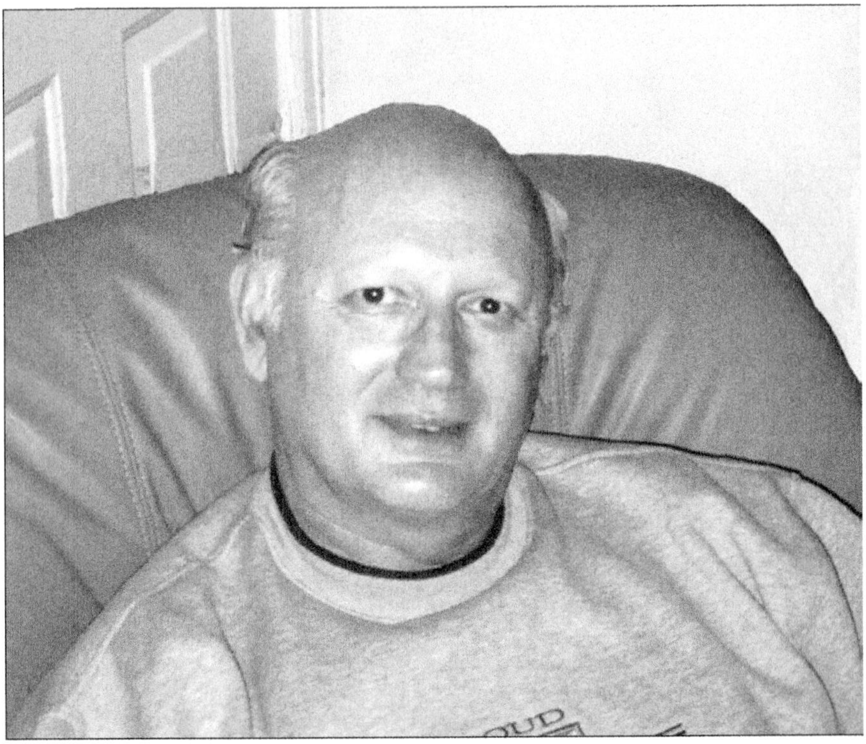

Paul Gabriel
What is your story?

What are 3 things that keep you going while you are in the pits?

Well, this is lately, but having gotten involved with the church, I pray. It helps a lot.

Then I think about all the good things in my life, like Connie, and the fun things that we are looking forward to in the future.

Those are three things...

What are 3 things you do to stay out of the pits?

The main thing is that I try not to focus on the negativity. That's the main thing, and so it's just a habit of thought. It can send you into a spiral of anger or depression, if you focus on all the bad things that are going on, or the scary things that could happen.

So I try and catch myself, when I find myself thinking or focusing on negative things. Then I try to turn it around consciously, and focus on the more positive things, or reframe it.

Another simple thing I do is get some exercise—take a walk. I find that a little exercise does surprisingly good things!

Connie and I do it too. We'll go out for a walk together. Even if I'm by myself at work, during the day, I'll just go out for a walk...

Then a third thing is to stay engaged in things I enjoy. An example is, I spend a lot of time working at the church. I do it because it energizes me, and I feel good.

Tell me something about your past—anything that comes to your mind.

What? **He chuckles...** Um, the biggest thing that's happened to me was getting separated from Peggy after 20-some years, you know.

It was kind of her idea to move out, but after a year or so, after I accepted it, I kind of enjoyed being by myself.

For her, it kind of backfired, in a sense, because I think her plan was to maybe force me to change and meet her goals.

It's like, well no, it's the best thing that happened to me. It gave me time to find out what I enjoy, and to be myself. I've changed tremendously! The last 5 years, or so, I've really been pretty happy, after a lifetime of being angry and depressed.

What happened to bring on your affliction?

It was depression. It was a funny thing. While getting separated and divorced, I think that's when I realized it was really depression. Then as I look back over my life, I think I have been depressed a good part of my life—even as a kid.

The awareness of that was a pretty big awareness! I think that some of it is even inherited, because I look back at my grandmother—who was a bitter angry person. That was depression. In those days, they didn't know what it was. I grew up around her, and I think it bleeds over into your life...

In my opinion, when I raised my attitude, it changed the physical chemicals in my brain. That made me stay up there.

I think if it is severe depression, it's something different. I don't know that it works that way, you know...

Then you look back, and wonder how could I have ever been that way?

I want to hear your story. For each of us has a different one... What makes you unique? What makes you the same?

What makes me unique is the circumstances of my life—who my parents were, and where I grew up. That's unique to me as a human being. No one can share in that. Good or bad, everyone is unique judging by their experiences.

What makes me the same is I am made of the same stuff as anyone else...

My personal belief is that we are all made of the same spirit. We're all identical. We just think we're different... In my opinion, the person that we are is not our experiences, we are really a spiritual being, and that's who I am.

Through the years, I grew and experienced more. Now I am in a much broader and wiser place—hopefully, after 56 years.

The experiences make me unique, because I don't think any one else experienced life exactly the way I experienced it.

What makes me the same is that I am in the world as a spiritual being, connected to everyone else. That makes me the same...

That was a difficult question! **Yah, People are afraid to make 'I' statements.**

How do you feel about where you are today?
What makes you happy?
What makes you sad?

Well, I feel great about where I am today! I'm very happy, and I attempt to not let other things make me happy or sad.

My personal belief is that teachings from the church are that being happy is a choice. It's a personal choice. It has nothing to do with what is going on around you. You can choose to be happy, even if your circumstances aren't so great.

I think that's true, so when I say things don't make me happy or sad, I don't think I'm there yet. It's a pretty high spiritual level.

There are things that make me happy. Having something to look forward to makes me happy. Connie makes me happy, and the kids make me happy—they also make me sad...

They weren't always on a good track, and now they are. So, they made me sad, and they now make me happy.

Now, I say, ok, I choose to be happy all the time—no matter what's going on around me, and I work to that goal. I mean, I'm not perfect, but that takes ownership over my own life.

Because I am happy more often than sad, I don't need my anti-depressants. I took them for about a year.

They kept me on the positive side longer, so that my brain actually generated more of the chemicals for a more uplifting life.

I have pretty much stayed there without the medication...

Do you have any regrets? If so, what are they?

Um, I try not to have any regrets, because, the best way to look at it is, well that's gone! It doesn't really matter anymore.

So, I try not to dwell too much on the past (although I do)...You know? You fall back on, "Oh I should've done this. I should've done that!" I should've been smarter! I should've been more successful!

So my biggest regret is that I have regrets! **We laugh...**

I guess that's kind of funny, but having regrets about the past is useless.

It's futile, and a waste of energy. So, knowing it intellectually is one thing, and actually putting it into practice, is something else.

What material thing really sings to you?

That's a hard one...

I think it would be my house— even though it's for sale. There's a lot of history there... So, the house deteriorated when I was down, and I started bringing my attitude and mental position up to a more positive level. The house is pretty nice now. It kind of reflects my mental state.

So the house, I think, is real important, and even though I'm selling it, I'm proud of how it is now. It's clean, and it's nice. It's comfortable. I could live there forever.

The reason I'm selling, is that I'm starting a new life with Connie, so... yah...

What are 2 interests you have?

I have a lot of interests, for sure. I like to read. I like to read about all sorts of things. I have been thinking about becoming a church practitioner. So I've been reading about metaphysics, and psychology, and things like that— Buddhism too...

I like what I'm doing at the church, like leading groups, and stuff like that.

So, I'm actually thinking about expanding that by going back to school to be a licensed counselor. It would be like a second career. It's very rewarding, too.

What would you say to God if He was standing right in front of you?

That's a pretty philosophical question, because I believe that God is not outside me, but inside me.

So if I saw God in front of me, I'd have to question what I was seeing! I see on the outside what is a reflection of the inside.

So, if I really thought it was God, it would be an expansion of what I see inside me.

For instance, in this belief I would say that if I have a perfect conscious level, when I look into someone's face, I would see the face of God.

So if a person looked in the mirror, they would see the face of God in their own face.
If I saw God, what I would say to God, I would also be saying it to myself.

I use to be a lot more tense. I was a little more fearful too. I was defensive and fearful. I'm a lot more comfortable with myself, so I don't snap at people. **I think you're having fun too.**

How long have you been afflicted with a mental illness?

I think I have had it my whole life! That year, I started realizing that I should not be feeling this way!

As I look back, I think my response was a depressed response.

Thirty years ago, people didn't even talk about mental illness! They didn't have a lot of knowledge about medication.

The degree of knowledge about depression today is phenomenal!

People's attitudes about mental illness are also much better!

So a person, like me, can say "Yah, I was depressed! It is a form of illness. There's no question about it!" I'm not ashamed to say that, so...
So there! **He chuckles.**

What makes your life worth living?

Meeting Connie, and my general attitude towards life, makes it an experience, and an adventure. Even when it gets tough, and things don't go your way, you really test that philosophy.

I consciously decide how I'll respond, rather than to react in certain pre-described ways.

If you feel a little bit of anger, you can act that way. I choose to act this way!

You know your hot buttons are, and to think through that, and say well no... It's one thing to philosophize, but it's another to put it into action. The earlier I catch that reaction, the easier it is to change it.

That's self awareness. Not that I'm perfect at it, but it's an amazing new way of being. **He chuckles a bit.**

If I choose to get a heart condition, because of the anger, that's my choice. I just choose not to do that anymore. It's not that I don't give a ----.

It's that I'm not going to get angry, and only hurt myself. It's a radical change and a way to look at life.

Where would you be without mental health support?

Well, I would be pretty miserable, probably.

I'll include the mental health support at the church I go to. Even if they're not mental health professionals, and don't want to be, they support you in the way a therapist would... I'm not a counselor per-say, but I'm in these groups to support you with acceptance.

So that, in itself, with the medication, was the lift I needed to change me. That's why I want to do practitioner work. It's life changing for people including myself!

The psychiatrist I went to said that I was not terribly depressed. I said, "Maybe not, but I am enough so that I'm not happy!"

He gave me a stronger dose of Zyban than I took to stop smoking. I hardly knew that I was taking it, but I would not slip into that depression. It just wouldn't let me go there.

It was great!

Knowing you, and the benefit of therapists and all the help you got, gave me the courage to go see this guy.

It seems like psychologists kind of go along with the fads, but Psychiatrists seem to be more factual, more scientific about their approach...

Seeing how much they helped you, gave me the courage to say, yah, this is a good thing!

Now, if you could tell the world your greatest dream, what would it be?

I have all kinds of dreams! You want fantasies or dreams? I'd like to see myself as a writer. I've always been interested in doing that. I enjoy doing it, but never sat down and done it.

I got an online course about writing. This lady's great! Some time I'll lend it to you. She teaches at NYU in New York. The whole first part of her course is you deciding what you want to write about.

She has a method, but it's really a meditation...

I saw Richard Bach one time, and he shared something amazing! He was walking down the street one day, and the book, "Jonathan Livingston Seagull", came to him all at once! He just transcribed what he had received. It was fabulous...

Summary:

Well, Paul, you surprised me! Your new way of life has softened your face, and your laugh is so delightful!

You have managed to find a reasonable amount of joy, peace, and love in the land of choices.

Some of your answers were quite unique, and they tell me that you have done a lot of inner work.

Because of this work, I see that you have begun to play and have fun. You appear to be full of a divine, playful spirit, and it shows...

I've known you for over 30 years, and did not know you wanted to be a writer! More power to you!

Your answer about regrets was very funny! You regret that you have regrets!

It is great having you back in our lives, and welcome to our home...

Dear World

It has been my honor to do these interviews. Each person has been quite special, and each has shared unselfishly.

Now that you have read our stories, and you have begun to, "Walk a Mile in Our Shoes", please take a moment to reflect and understand.

We are people who struggle - just like you.

We have good and bad days - same as you.

We cry and laugh - like you also.

Yet, many of us need extra medical assistance to give quality to our lives.

Let me share a challenge that we face. My therapist concurred that treatment at publicly funded, community mental health centers, has been drastically reduced.

I've heard that people call less often, make shorter calls, and wait longer for their calls to be answered.

Case loads of some mental health experts have doubled!

Though professionals at these centers have been affected, they are still caring and efficient. Yet, they can only spread themselves so far...

I believe mental illness has affected everyone on this planet in one way or another.

So, let's treat each other as equals. We are all deserving of this, by nature of our humanity...

My hope would be, for all of us, to help those who need care, especially when they cannot speak for themselves...

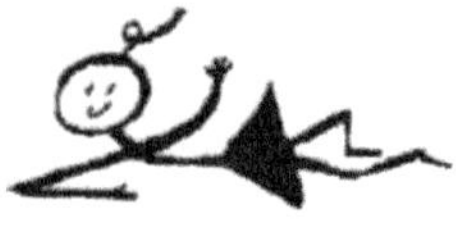

Printed in Dunstable, United Kingdom

91218263R00167